# Pediatric Spots

# Pediatric Spots


**Saad Saleh Al Ani**

MBChB, CAB Ped, IBCLC

Professor of Pediatric
Senior Pediatric Consultant
Head, Pediatric Department
Khorfakkan Hospital
Sharjah Medical District
Ministry of Health, UAE


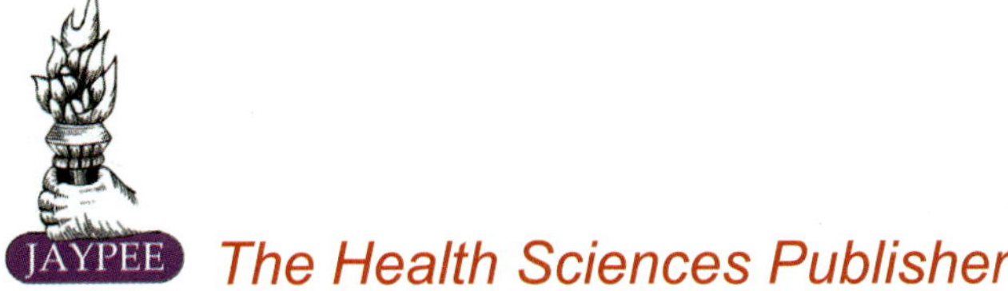


JAYPEE *The Health Sciences Publisher*

New Delhi | London | Philadelphia | Panama

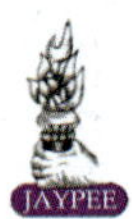

**Jaypee Brothers Medical Publishers (P) Ltd**

### Headquarters

Jaypee Brothers Medical Publishers (P) Ltd
4838/24, Ansari Road, Daryaganj
New Delhi 110 002, India
Phone: +91-11-43574357
Fax: +91-11-43574314
**Email: jaypee@jaypeebrothers.com**

### Overseas Offices

J.P. Medical Ltd
83 Victoria Street, London
SW1H 0HW (UK)
Phone: +44 20 3170 8910
Fax: +44 (0)20 3008 6180
Email: info@jpmedpub.com

Jaypee Medical Inc
The Bourse
111 South Independence Mall East
Suite 835, Philadelphia, PA 19106, USA
Phone: +1 267-519-9789
Email: jpmed.us@gmail.com

Jaypee Brothers Medical Publishers (P) Ltd
Bhotahity, Kathmandu, Nepal
Phone: +977-9741283608
Email: kathmandu@jaypeebrothers.com

Jaypee-Highlights Medical Publishers Inc
City of Knowledge, Bld. 237, Clayton
Panama City, Panama
Phone: +1 507-301-0496
Fax: +1 507-301-0499
Email: cservice@jphmedical.com

Jaypee Brothers Medical Publishers (P) Ltd
17/1-B Babar Road, Block-B, Shaymali
Mohammadpur, Dhaka-1207
Bangladesh
Mobile: +08801912003485
Email: jaypeedhaka@gmail.com

Website: www.jaypeebrothers.com
Website: www.jaypeedigital.com

© 2016, Jaypee Brothers Medical Publishers



*Pediatric Spots*

*First Edition*: **2016**

ISBN 978-93-5152-931-6

*Printed at* Sanat Printers

## PREFACE

As pediatric science is growing and various new researches are introduced, specially for those preparing their postgraduate study in pediatrics, family medicine, general practice and those who treat children during their daily clinic, so this book is useful to understand and memorize them to use efficiently in their study. This is designed and prepared with the purpose to help them in a simple and smooth way.

I hope this book will help them to get the desired benefit, and to build their knowledge and skills and to step up in their ways to progress.

**Saad Saleh Al Ani**

_________________ **CONTENTS** _________________

# Accidents and Emergency

## 1.1. Estimate the Bruise's Age by Color

| Time | Color | Variations in color |
|---|---|---|
| <1 day | Red | Red to reddishblue |
| Day 1– 4 | Blue | Dark blue to purple |
| Day 5–7 | Green | Green to yellow-green |
| Day 7–10 | Yellow | Yellow to brown |
| Week 1–3 | Normal | |

## 1.2. Causes of Miosis Include {(CO) 2P3S}

1. Cholinergics and clonidine
2. Opiates and organophosphates
3. Phencyclidine, phenothiazine and pilocarpine
4. Sedatives (barbiturates).

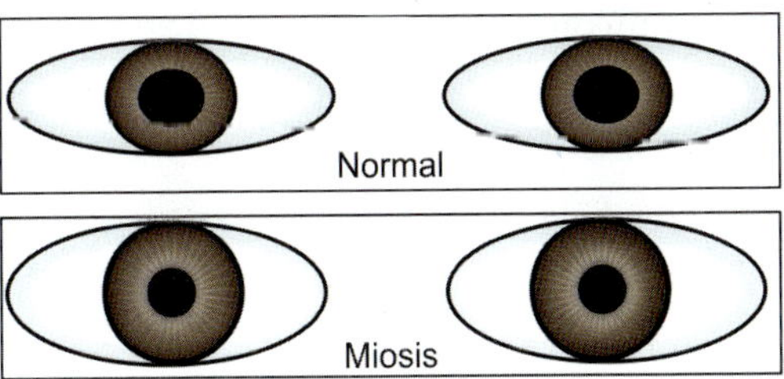


**Fig. 1.1**: Miosis vs. normal pupil

## 1.3. Causes of Mydriasis Include (AAAS)

1. Anticholinergics (atropine)
2. Antihistamines
3. Antidepressants (cyclic)
4. Sympathomimetics (amphetamine, cocaine and LSD).

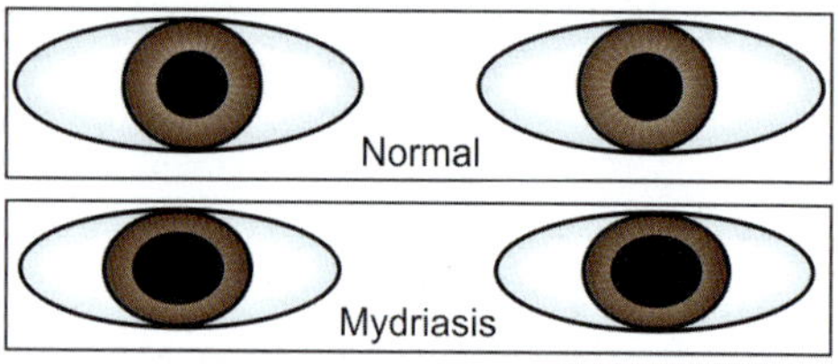

**Fig. 1.2**: Mydriasis vs. normal pupil

## 1.4. Causes of Diaphoretic Skin (SOAP)

1. Sympathomimetics
2. Organophosphates
3. Aspirin (salicylates)
4. PCP (phencyclidine).

## 1.5. Causes of Red Skin

1. Carbon monoxide
2. Boric acid.

## 1.6. Causes of Blue Skin

1. Cyanosis
2. Methemoglobinemia.

## 1.7. Activated Charcoal is Ineffective or Contraindicated in the Following: (CHEMICAL CamP)

- Caustics
- Hydrocarbons
- Electrolytes (common ones)
- Metals
- Iron
- Cyanide
- Alcohols
- Lithium
- Camphor
- Phosphorus.

## 1.8. The Symptoms of Acetaminophen Overdose Occur in Four Stages

**N.B:**
1. With overdoses, glutathione stores are overwhelmed and toxic metabolites accumulate.
2. An acute toxic dose in a child <12 years of age is about 150 mg/kg and in adolescents and adult it is ~ 15 gm.

| Stage | Time | Symptoms |
|---|---|---|
| 1 | 0–24 hours | If any signs, nausea, vomiting, normal liver function tests (LFTs) |
| 2 | 24–48 hours | Asymptomatic; may be RUQ pain; LFTs may begin to increase |
| 3 | 48–96 hours | Peak of symptoms; AST≥20,000, prolonged PT, death from hepatic failure or coagulopathy |
| 4 | 4–14 days | Recovery or death; symptoms resolve in survivors |

## 1.9. Symptoms of Anticholinergics Overdose

### 1.9.1. Anticholinergic agents include

1. Some antihistamines (diphenhydramine)
2. Antidepressants (amitriptyline and imipramine)
3. Antispasmodics
4. Antiparkinson agents
5. Atropine
6. Toxic plants (mushrooms, jimson weed and deadly nightshade).

### 1. 9.2. The symptoms are key

- Dry as a bone: ↓ Sweating and ↓ urine output
- Red as a beet: Flushing
- Blind as a bat: Mydriasis
- Mad as a hatter: Agitation and seizure
- Hot as a hare : Hyperthermia.

## 1.10.  The Symptoms of Iron Overdose

### 1.10.1.  There are 5 phases of iron toxicity

1. GI stage (30 minutes to 6 hours)
   - Nausea, vomiting, diarrhea and abdominal pain
   - Hematemesis and bloody diarrhea in severe cases
   - Symptoms are due to the direct damage to the GI and intestinal mucosa.
2. Stability (6–24 hours)
3. Systemic toxicity (within 48 hours)
   - Hypovolemic shock
   - Cardiovascular  collapse
   - Severe metabolic acidosis (positive anion gap).

4.  Hepatotoxicity (2–3 days postingestion)
    • Hepatic failure
    • Coagulation disruption worsen GI bleeding.
5.  GI/pyloric scarring (2–5 weeks postingestion).

## 1.10.2. An elemental iron ingestion of

•  20 mg/kg : Mild
•  40 mg/kg : Moderate
•  >60 mg/kg : Severe.

## 1.11.  Opiate Overdose

### 1.11.1.  Common opiates include: ( M3PHC) n

•  Morphine
•  Propoxyphene
•  Methadone
•  Heroin
•  Mepridine
•  Codeine.

### 1.11.2.  The classic triad of

1.  Coma
2.  Respiratory depression
3.  Pinpoint pupils (miosis).

### 1.11.3. Other expected findings of opiate overdose

1.  Analgesia
2.  Altered mood
3.  GI issues
4.  Decreased GI motility
5.  Nausea and vomiting
6.  Abdominal pain (increased colonic and biliary tone)
7.  Increased anal sphincter tone.

## 1.12. Salicylates Poisoning

### 1.12.1. Three systems are affected

1.  GI: (nausea and vomiting)
2.  Respiratory:(hyperpnea leading to respiratory alkalosis)
3.  CNS: (if severe) (agitation, confusion and coma).

## 1.12.2. Salicylate level

> 30 mg/dL is potentially toxic
> 40 mg/dL is usually symptomatic
> 100 mg/dL  signifies serious toxicity.

## 1.13.  Theophylline Overdose

- Leads to the following electrolyte abnormalities which are common:
  ↑ Glucose and calcium
  ↓ Potassium and phosphate.
  Metabolic acidosis.

## 1.14.  Tricyclic Antidepressant Ingestion

- They inhibit cardiac fast sodium channels
- Symptoms occur within 30 minutes to 6 hours
- Ingestion of 10–20 mg/kg is moderate to serious.

## 1.14.1. CNS effects are more prominent in children and include

1. Drowsiness
2. Lethargy
3. Seizures
4. Coma
5. Cardiac effects are:
   - Tachycardia
   - Hypertension or hypotension
   - Widened QRS
   - Prolonged QT.

## 1.14.2. Be aware of CCCA in tricyclic antidepressants

- Coma
- Convulsions
- Cardiac arrhythmias
- Acidosis.

## 1.15. Caustic Substance Ingestion

These fall into either alkaline or acidic agents.

## 1.15.1. Alkaline agents and characteristic

Bleach, ammonia, cleaners for ovens and drains, automatic dishes washer detergent, hair relaxers and lye
- Tasteless

- Cause severe, deep and liquefaction necrosis
- May lead to scar tissue with stricture.

## 1.15.2. Acidic agents and characteristics

Toilet bowl cleaner, grout cleaner, rust remover, automotive battery liquids and metal cleaners
- Bitter taste.
- Coagulation necrosis (superficial).
- May lead to thick eschar formation, severe gastritis, metabolic acidosis, or acute renal failure.

For caustic substance ingestion do not:
- Neutralize
- Induce emesis
- Do gastric lavage
- Give activated charcoal.

## 1.16. Ethanol Ingestion

### 1.16.1. Signs and symptoms of ethanol ingestion include

1. CNS disturbances:
   - Depression (slurred speech, ataxia and stupor to coma)
   - Seizure.
2. Respiratory depression
3. GI disturbance:
   - Nausea
   - Vomiting.
4. Hypothermia
5. Hypoglycemia.

### 1.16.2. A high osmolal gap should make one suspicious for ingestion of

1. Ethanol
2. Methanol
3. Ethylene glycol
4. Isopropyl alcohol.

## 1.17. Methanol Ingestion

### 1.17.1. Symptoms

- Initial nonspecific complaints:
  - Malaise
  - Headache

- – Abdominal discomfort
- – Nausea
- – Vomiting.
- • 24 hours later, the child will develop:
  - – Visual disturbances with blurry vision and photophobia
  - – Optic nerve damage leading to blindness
  - – CNS depression
  - – Severe metabolic acidosis (high anion gap)    .

## 1.17.2. Look for triad of

1. Visual complaints
2. Abdominal pain
3. Metabolic acidosis (without lactic acidosis or ketonuria).

## 1.18. Ethylene Glycol Ingestion

### 1.18.1. There are 3 stages of intoxication

Stage 1: (1–12 hours)
- • Appear drunk with nausea and vomiting
- • Drowsiness
- • Slurred speech
- • Lethargy.

Stage 2: (12–36 hours)
- • Respiratory problems—Tachypnea
- • Cyanosis
- • Pulmonary edema
- • ARDS
- • Death can occur.

Stage 3: (2–3 days)
- • Cardiac failure
- • Seizures
- • Cerebral edema
- • Renal failure.

### 1.18.2. Like methanol, ethylene glycol ingestion leads to

- • Metabolic acidosis (without lactic acidosis or ketonuria)
- • High osmolal gap.

## 1.19. Organophosphate Ingestion

### 1.19.1. Inhibition of cholinesterase leads to the cholinergic toxidrome (DUMBELS) (N.B. there is increased secretions)

- Diarrhea
- Urination
- Miosis (pinpoint)
- Bronchorrhea/bronchospasm
- Emesis
- Lacrimation
- Salivation.

## 1.20. Hydrocarbon Ingestion

### 1.20.1. The clinical findings include

- Coughing
- Chocking
- Gagging
- Wheezing
- Severe respiratory distress
- Mild CNS depression
- Fever.

## 1.21. Burn

### 1.21.1. Classification of burn

- First-degree (superficial)
  - Red, dry, minor swelling and pain
  - They generally resolve in 5–7 days.
- Second-degree (partial thickness)
  - Red, wet, very painful, often with blisters or blebs
  - The tissue underneath is still well-perfused
  - It may take 2–5 weeks for these to heal.
- Third-degree (full thickness)
  - Dry, leathery, waxy and have no pain associated with them.
  - They require grafting to large areas or healing from edges in smaller areas.

### 1.21.2. Measurement of burn areas follows the rule of nines (>14 years old)

| | |
|---|---|
| • Head and neck | 9% |
| • Each upper limb | 9% |
| • Thorax and abdomen—Front | 18% |
| • Thorax and abdomen—Back | 18% |
| • Perineum | 1% |
| • Each lower limb | 18% |

### 1.21.3. Rule of Palm (<10 years of age)

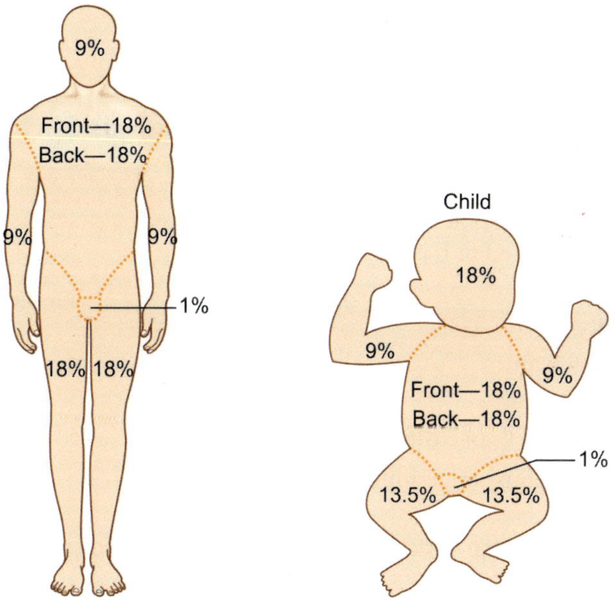


**Fig. 1.3**: Percentage of burn areas in a child vs. adult

- Child's palm not including fingers = 0.5–1% body surface area
- Useful in smaller burns.

## 1.22. Head Injury

### 1.22.1. Physical findings indicating more serious injury include

1. Scalp swelling or step-off
2. Basilar skull fracture (often associated with CSF leak and cranial nerve damage):
   - Raccoon eyes
   - Battle sign
   - Hemotympanum.
3. Temporal bone fracture
   - Bleeding from the external auditory canal
   - CSF otorrhea
   - Hearing loss
   - Facial paralysis.
4. Papillary changes, papillededma doesn't develop immediately
5. Infants:
   - Retinal hemorrhages (abuse)
   - Other bruises.

### 1.22.2. When to definitely order a CT scan (high-risk) in head injury

- Depressed mental status
- Focal neurological signs
- Signs of depressed or basilar skill fracture
- Seizure
- Irritability
- Acute skull feature
- Bulging fontanel
- Vomiting more than 5 times or for > 6 hours
- Loss of consciousness > 1 minute.

### 1.22.3. Intermediate-risk patients who have the followings

- Loss of consciousness < 1 minute.
- Vomiting 3 – 4 times.
- Lethargy or irritability now resolved.
- Behavioral changes.
- Mechanism: High force, fall onto a hard surface, or unknown, unwitnessed and vague.
- Hematoma, and specially large or nonfrontal.
- Nonacute skull fracture.

### 1.22.4. When to discharge with instruction (low-risk)

- Mechanism of injury is low energy (e.g. fall of <3ft)
- No signs or symptoms
- No loss of consciousness.

### 1.22.5. Concussion grades

| Grade | Confusion | Amnesia | Loss of consciousness |
|-------|-----------|---------|-----------------------|
| I | Yes | No | No |
| II | Yes | Yes | No |
| III | Yes | Yes | Yes |

### 1.22.6. Concussion and time before return to contact sports

| | Minimum time to return to play | Time asymptomatic |
|-----|-------------------------------|-------------------|
| I | 20 minutes | At the initial exam |
| II | 1 week | 1 week |
| III | 1 month | 1week |

## 1.23. Grade of Ankle Sprains

| | Grade I (mild) | Grade II (moderate) | Grade III (severe) |
|-----------------|----------------|---------------------|---------------------|
| Swelling | Mild | Moderate | Severe |
| Tenderness | Mild | Moderate | Severe |
| Loss of function | Minimal | Difficult to ambulate | Unable to bear weight |
| Treatment | 7–10 days rest | 2–4 weeks rest | 5–10 weeks rest |

## Bibliography

1. http://publications.nice.org.uk/head-injury-cg56/guidance.
2. McNeil consumer and specialty pharmaceuticals. Guidelines for the management of Acetaminophen overdose. 7050 Camp Hill Road. Fort Washington, PA 19034.
3. Schwartz AJ, Ricci LR. How Accurately Can Bruises Be Aged in Abused Children? http://pediatrics.aappublications.org/content/97/2/254.

## 2.1. ECG Findings

### 2.1.1. Nomenclature of electrocardiogram (ECG) waves and intervals

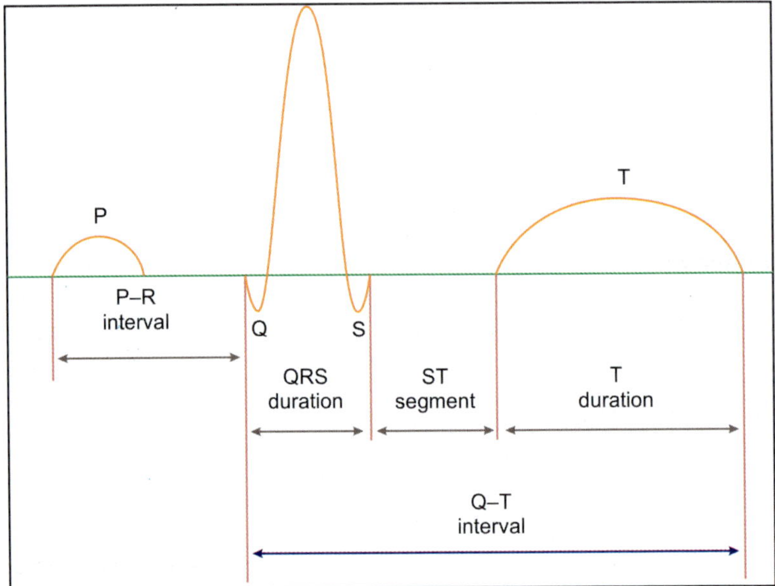


**Fig. 2.1**: Nomenclature of ECG waves and intervals

### 2.1.2. Important intervals

#### 2.1.2.1. P–R interval

**P–R interval**
- Indicates the time between atrial and ventricular depolarization.
- It is a reflection of mostly AV node conduction.
- Normal duration is 3–5 small squares (120–200 ms), because a "small square" is defined as 40 ms).
- A P–R interval longer than 200 ms (1 big square) in teens and adults, is the definition of 1° AV block.

- Intervals shorter than 120 ms (3 small squares) in teens and adults may indicate:
  1. Wolff-Parkinson-White (WPW) (short interval with delta wave)
  2. Junctional rhythm (with retrograde P wave)
  3. Left atrial overload (widened P wave).

### 2.1.2.2. QRS duration

**QRS duration**
- It is usually < 100 ms (½ a big square).

**QRS >120 ms may be caused by**
- Bundle branch block (BBB) (right or left)
- Ectopic ventricular beat (PVC)
- Ventricular rhythm
- Ventricular pacemaker
- Drugs that prolong conduction (e.g. tricyclics)
- WPW
- Electrolyte problems (hyperkalemia).

### 2.1.2.3. Q–T interval

**Q–T interval**
- Varies with heart rate.
- The corrected Q–T interval (QTc) for heart rate is normally 340–440 ms.

**With prolonged QTc there is  a tendency to develop:**
- Recurrent syncope
- Sudden death
- Torsades de pointes.

**Causes of prolonged QTc:**
- Genetic or congenital prolonged QT syndrome (in a child without medications).
- Long QT + sensorineural deafness = Jervell and Lange-Nielsen syndrome.

**Other etiologies for prolonged Q–T interval include:**
- Tricyclic overdose (specially in adolescent)
- Hypocalcemia
- Hypomagnesemia
- Hypokalemia
- Type $I_a$ and III antiarrhythmics
- ($I_a$ = quinidine, procainamide; III = amiodarone, sotalol)
- Starvation with electrolyte abnormalities
- CNS insult.

**Short QTc may be caused by:**
- Hypercalcemia
- Digitalis
- Congenital.

## 2.1.3. Waveforms and segments

### 2.1.3.1. P wave

**P wave:**
- Originating in sinus node (SA)
- Result from the depolarization of the atrium
- Normal P wave
  - 2 mm in height
  - <120 ms (3 small squares) in duration
  - The axis is 0–+90°
- Most information from P wave can be derived from lead II, aVR and $V_1$
- The normal P wave is:
  - Positive in lead I, II and aVF
  - Positive or biphasic in $V_1$
  - Negative in aVR.

**A retrograde P wave:**
- Originating outside the SA node
- It is negative in II (and II and aVF)
- It is positive in aVR
- Indicating an ectopic focus which is originating in:
  1. Inferior part of the atrium
  2. The AV junction (often results in short P–R interval).

**Right atrial preponderance:**
(enlargement, hypertrophy and overload)
- The P wave width stays normal (<120 ms)
- Peaking of P wave in lead II and $V_1$.

**Left atrial overload:**
- Widened, notched "M" shaped P wave in lead II
- Decreased P waves amplitude is seen in severe hyperkalemia.

### 2.1.3.2. T wave

**T wave**
- Typically positive in $V_1$ at birth → age 7 days then inverted.
- Should remain inverted in $V_1$ until ages 9–10 years.
- They may be either inverted or upright in $V_1$ during teen years.
- If T wave remain positive after 7 days and upto 10 years of age in $V_1$, this may indicate right ventricular hypertrophy.

**Peaked T waves can occur with:**
- Hyperkalemia
- Intracerebral hemorrhage.

### 2.1.3.3. U wave

**U wave**
- Usually small occurs just after T wave
- It is mainly something to look at in older adolescents or adults
- Best seen in $V_2$–$V_3$
- Usually a < 1 mm, rounded deflection in the same direction of T wave.

**Prominent U wave**
- An increased tendency for *torsades de pointes*
- It is seen with:
  - Hypokalemia
  - Bradycardia
  - Digitalis
  - Amiodarone.

### 2.1.3.4. ST segment

- There are 3 main causes of ST segment elevation. These are:
  1. Acute MI
  2. Prinzmetal's angina
  3. Pericarditis.
- The first 2 are almost never seen in children.
- Pericarditis is the most common cause of cardiac chest pain in pediatrics and it affects the whole heart, so ST changes should be seen in most leads.

**ST segment elevation may also seen in:**
- Early repolarization variant
- Intracerebral hemorrhage
- Hypertrophic cardiomyopathy
- LVH

- LBBB
- Cocaine abuse
- Myocarditis
- Hypothermia.

**ST segment depression occurs in pediatrics with:**
- Subendocardial ischemia (specially if down-sloping or flat).
- LVH with strain (ST depression with flipped T wave in left precordial leads).
- RVH (cause RAD, ST segment depression preceding a flipped T wave in $V_1$).
- Digitalis effect.
- Hypokalemia.

### *2.1.3.5. QRS complex*

**QRS complex: 1**
- Depolarization of the ventricles occurs simultaneously after the depolarization of the interventricular septum.
- The mean vector of depolarization of the interventricular septum points from patient's left to right, across septum.

**QRS complex: 2**
- A small, initial deflection, which is positive in $V_1$ (R wave) and negative in $V_6$ (Q wave).
- A septal Q wave in $V_6$ generally means normal initial depolarization.
- The mean QRS vector is strongly to the patient's left so a large negative deflection in $V_1$ and positive deflection in $V_6$.

**QRS complex: 3**
- On the frontal plane, the mean vector is –30 to +100°
- The normal duration of the QRS is < 120 ms.

## 2.1.4. Features of the normal and abnormal rhythms

### *2.1.4.1. Normal sinus rhythm*

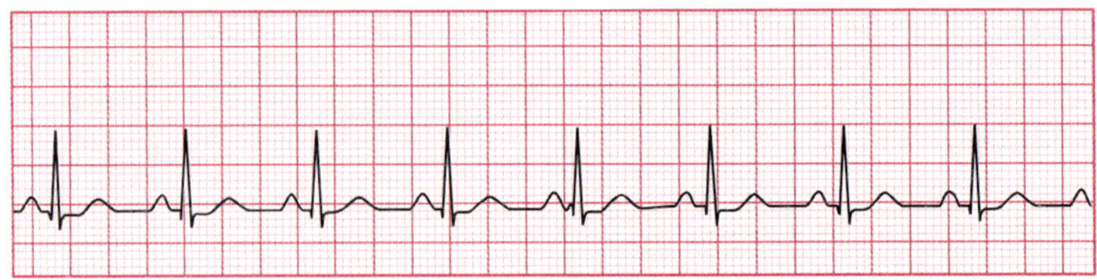

**Fig. 2.2**: Normal sinus rhythm

- Rhythm—Regular.
- Rate—(60–100 bpm).
- QRS duration—Normal.
- P wave—Visible before each QRS complex.
- P–R interval—Normal (<5 small squares. Anything above and this would be 1st degree block).
- Indicates that the electrical signal is generated by the sinus node and traveling in a normal fashion in the heart.

### 2.1.4.2. Sinus bradycardia

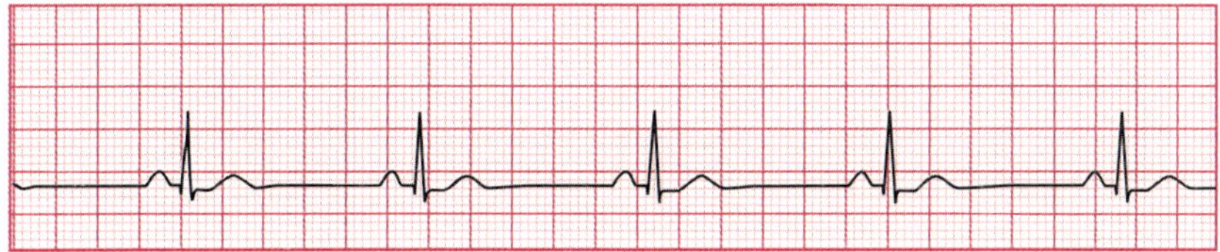

**Fig. 2.3**: Sinus bradycardia

- Rhythm—Regular
- Rate—Less than 60 beats per minute
- QRS duration—Normal
- P wave—Visible before each QRS complex
- P–R interval—Normal
- Usually benign and often caused by patients on β-blockers.

### 2.1.4.3. Sinus tachycardia

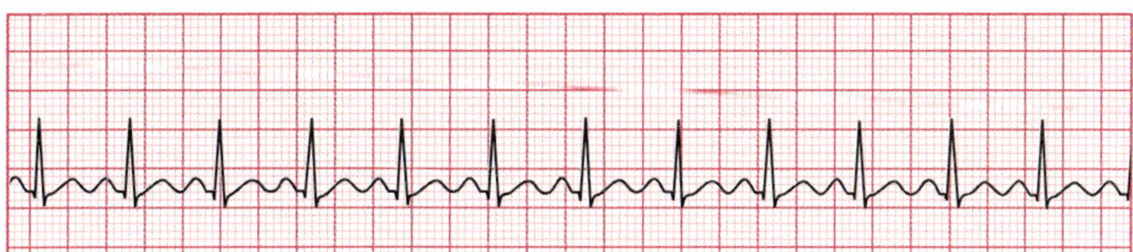

**Fig. 2.4**: Sinus tachycardia

- Rhythm—Regular
- Rate—More than 100 beats per minute
- QRS duration—Normal
- P wave—Visible before each QRS complex
- P–R interval—Normal
- The impulse generating the heartbeats are normal, but they are occurring at a faster pace than normal. Seen during exercise.

### *2.1.4.4. Supraventricular tachycardia (SVT) abnormal*

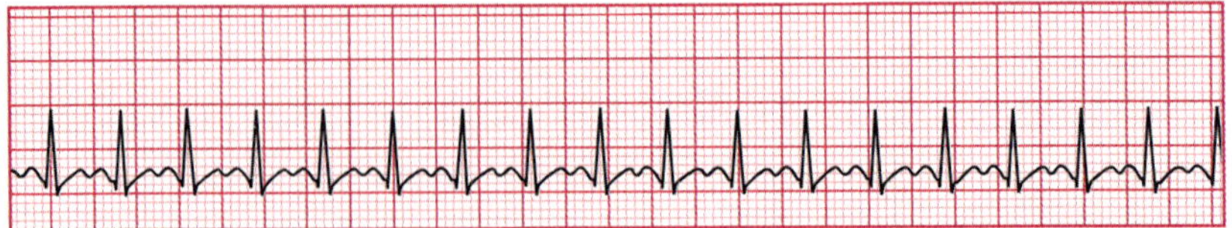

**Fig. 2.5**: Abnormal supraventricular tachycardia

- Rhythm—Regular.
- Rate—140–220 beats per minute.
- QRS duration—Usually normal.
- P wave—Often buried in preceding T wave.
- P–R interval—Depends on site of supraventricular pacemaker.
- Impulses stimulating the heart are not being generated by the sinus node, but instead are coming from a collection of tissue around and involving the atrioventricular (AV) node.

### *2.1.4.5. Atrial fibrillation*

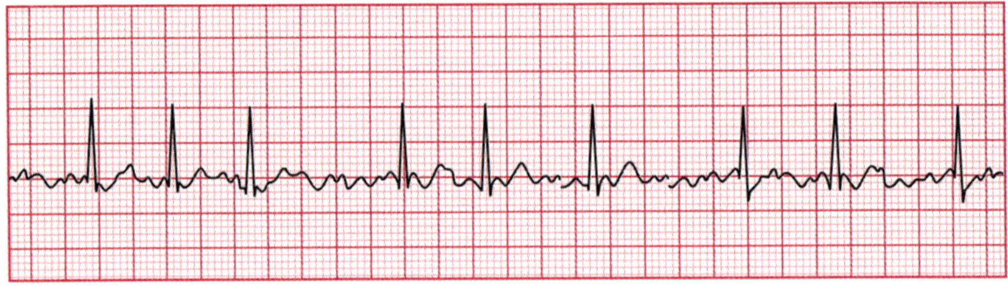

**Fig. 2.6**: Atrial fibrillation

- Rhythm—Irregularly irregular.
- Rate—Usually 100–160 beats per minute but slower if on medication.
- QRS duration—Usually normal.
- P wave—Not distinguishable as the atria are firing off all over.
- P–R interval—Not measurable.
- The atria fire electrical impulses in an irregular fashion causing irregular heart rhythm.

### *2.1.4.6. Atrial flutter*

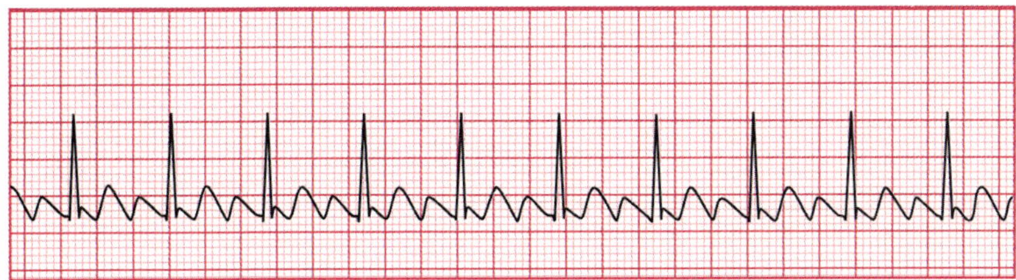

**Fig. 2.7**: Atrial flutter

- Rhythm—Regular.
- Rate—Around 110 beats per minute.
- QRS duration—Usually normal.
- P wave—Replaced with multiple F (flutter) waves, usually at a ratio of 2:1 (2F-1QRS) but sometimes 3:1.
- P wave rate—300 beats per minute.
- P–R interval—Not measurable.
- As with SVT the abnormal tissue generating the rapid heart rate is also in the atria, however, the atrioventricular node is not involved in this case.

### *2.1.4.7. First degree AV block*

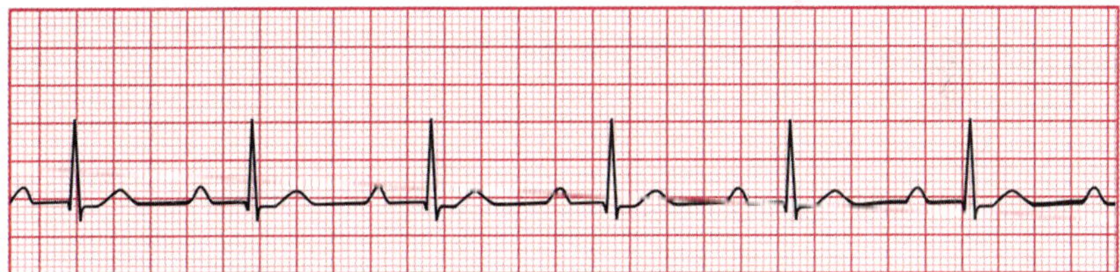

**Fig. 2.8**: First degree AV block

- Rhythm—Regular
- Rate—Normal
- QRS duration—Normal
- P wave—Ratio 1:1
- P wave rate—Normal
- P–R interval—Prolonged (>5 small squares).

### *2.1.4.8. Second degree AV block type I (Wenckebach)*

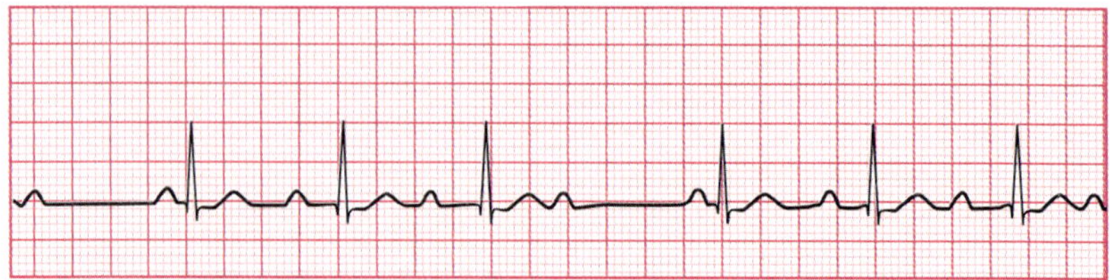

**Fig. 2.9**: Second degree AV block type I (Wenckebach)

- Rhythm—Regularly irregular.
- Rate—Normal or slow.
- QRS duration—Normal.
- P wave—Ratio 1:1 for 2, 3 or 4 cycles then 1:0.
- P wave rate—Normal but faster than QRS rate.
- P–R interval—Progressive lengthening of P–R interval until a QRS complex is dropped.

### *2.1.4.9. Second degree AV block type II*

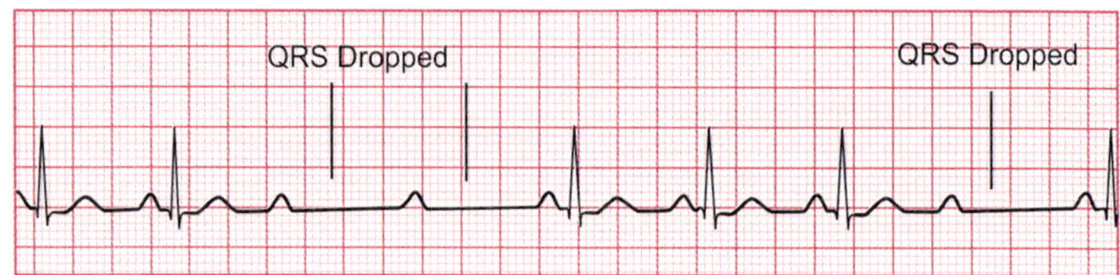


**Fig. 2.10**: Second degree AV block type II

- Rhythm—Regular
- Rate—Normal or slow
- QRS duration—Prolonged
- P wave—Ratio 2:1, 3:1
- P wave rate—Normal but faster than QRS rate
- P–R interval—Normal or prolonged but constant.

## *2.1.4.10. Third degree heart block*

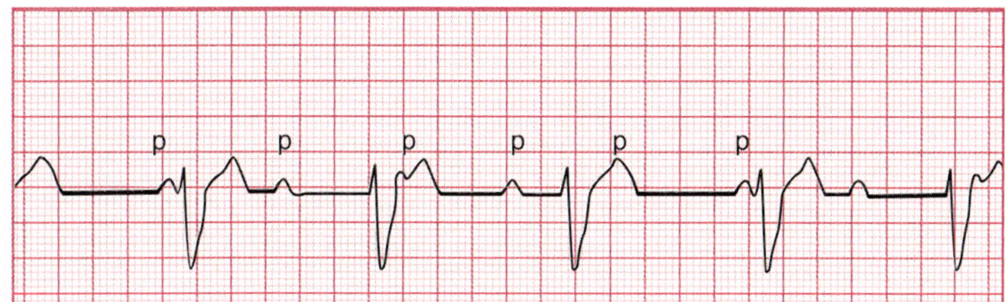

**Fig. 2.11**: Third degree heart block

- Rhythm—Regular.
- Rate—Slow.
- QRS duration—Prolonged.
- P wave—Unrelated.
- P wave rate—Normal but faster than QRS rate.
- P-R interval—Variation.
- Complete AV block—No atrial impulses pass through the atrioventricular node and the ventricles generate their own rhythm.

## *2.1.4.11. Bundle branch block*

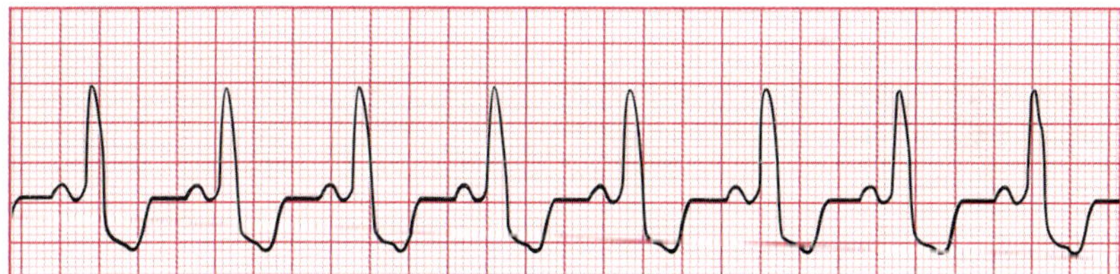

**Fig. 2.12**: Bundle branch block

- Rhythm—Regular
- Rate—Normal
- QRS duration—Prolonged
- P wave—Ratio 1:1
- P wave rate—Normal and same as QRS rate
- P-R interval—Normal.

### 2.1.4.12. Premature ventricular complexes

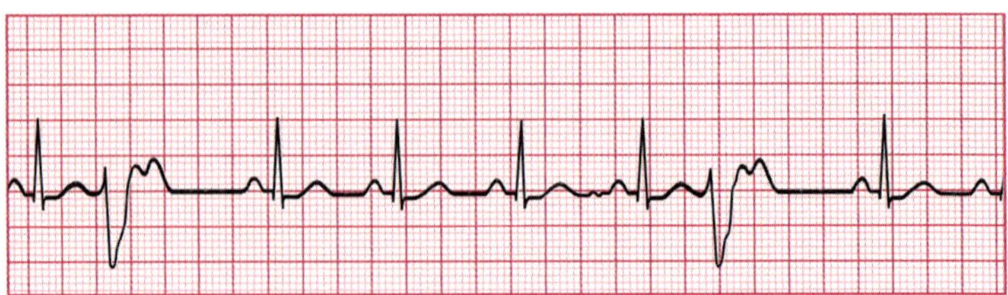

**Fig. 2.13**: Premature ventricular complexes

- Rhythm—Regular.
- Rate—Normal.
- QRS duration—Normal.
- P wave—Ratio 1:1.
- P wave rate—Normal and same as QRS rate.
- P-R interval—Normal.
- Also you'll see 2 odd waveforms, these are the ventricles depolarizing prematurely in response to a signal within the ventricles. (Above—Unifocal PVC's as they look alike if they differed in appearance they would be called multifocal PVC's, as below).

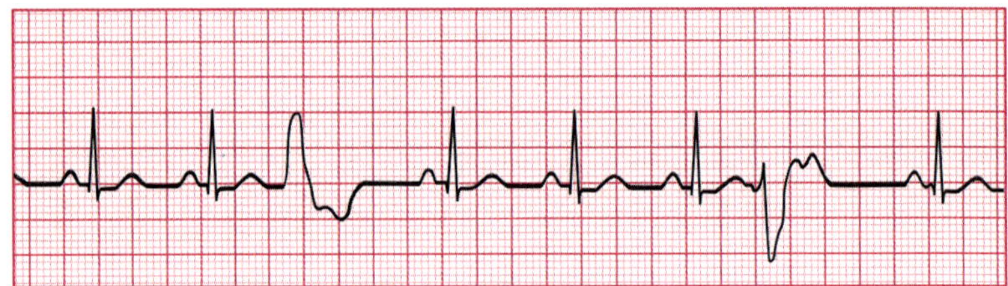

**Fig. 2.14**: Multifocal PVC's

### 2.1.4.13. Junctional rhythms

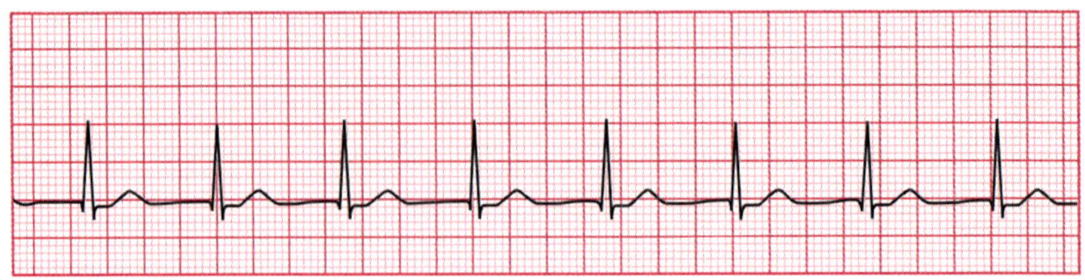

**Fig. 2.15**: Junctional rhythms

- Rhythm—Regular
- Rate—40-60 beats per minute
- QRS duration—Normal
- P wave—Ratio 1:1 if visible. Inverted in lead II
- P wave rate—Same as QRS rate
- P–R interval—Variable.

### 2.1.4.13.1. Accelerated junctional rhythm

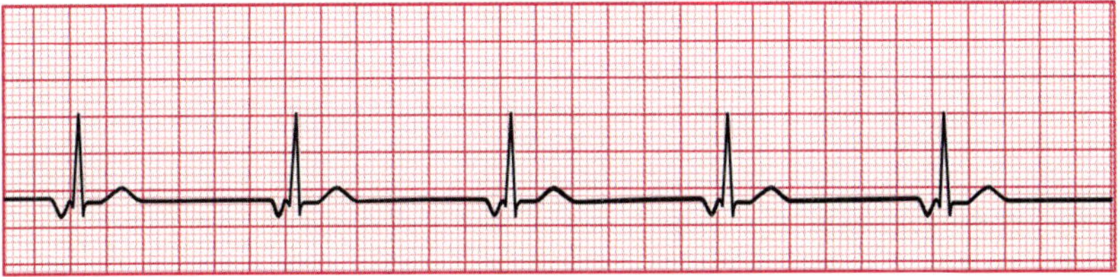

**Fig. 2.16**: Accelerated junctional rhythm

### 2.1.4.14. Ventricular tachycardia (VT) abnormal

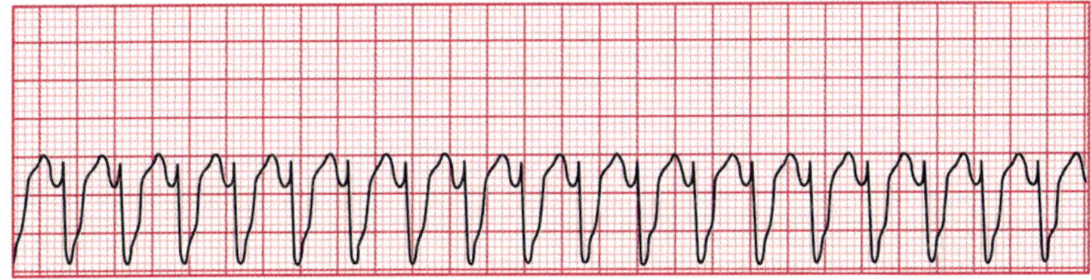

**Fig. 2.17**: Ventricular tachycardia

- Rhythm—Regular.
- Rate—180-190 beats per minute.
- QRS duration—Prolonged.
- P wave—Not seen.
- Results from abnormal tissues in the ventricles generating.
- A rapid and irregular heart rhythm. Poor cardiac output is usually associated with this rhythm thus causing cardiac arrest. Shock this rhythm if the patient is unconscious and without a pulse.

### 2.1.4.15. *Ventricular tachycardia (VT) abnormal*

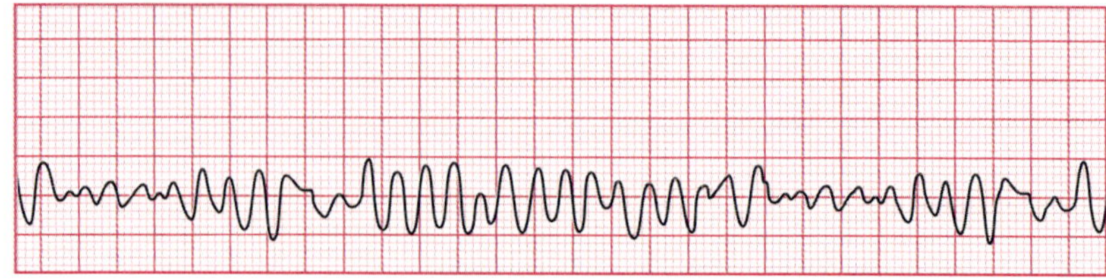

**Fig. 2.18**: Abnormal ventricular tachycardia

- Rhythm—Irregular
- Rate—300+, disorganized
- QRS duration—Not recognizable
- P wave—Not seen
- This patient needs to be defibrillated!! QUICKLY.

### 2.1.4.16. *Asystole—Abnormal*

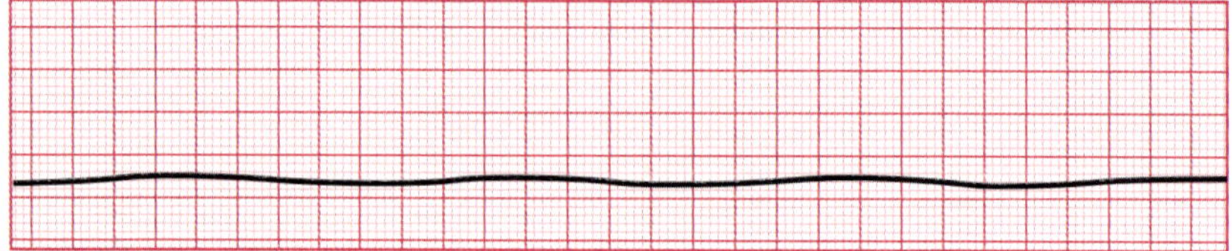

**Fig. 2.19**: Asystole

- Rhythm—Flat
- Rate—0 beats per minute
- QRS duration—None
- P wave—None
- Carry out CPR!!

### 2.1.4.17. *Myocardial infarct (MI)*

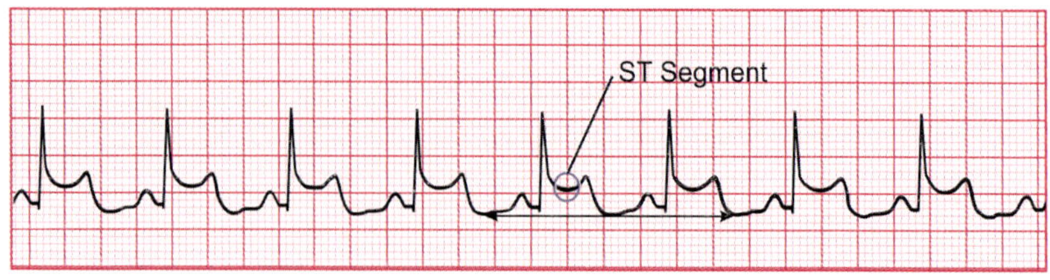


**Fig. 2.20**: Myocardial infarction

- Rhythm—Regular
- Rate—80 beats per minute
- QRS duration—Normal
- P wave—Normal
- ST element does not go isoelectric which indicates infarction.

## 2.1.5 Ventricular hypertrophy

### *2.1.5.1. Left ventricular hypertrophy (LVH)*

1. LVH is age-dependent
   A negative T wave in lead $V_6$ after 7 days of life, think of LVH.
2. • In infancy: The mean QRS being moved to the left and posteriorly
   • In frontal plane, the QRS axis may move to 0–60°; <30° in an infant is very uncommon and suggests LVH.
3. • Without an axis shift, the diagnosis of LVH is based on voltage criteria:
   – R waves less than 5th percentile or S waves more than 95th percentile in $V_3R$ and $V_1$
   – R waves more than 96th percentile in $V_5$ and $V_6$.
4. • In older adolescents: LVH causes an exaggerated:
   – Negative deflection in $V_1$
   – Positive deflection in $V_6$.

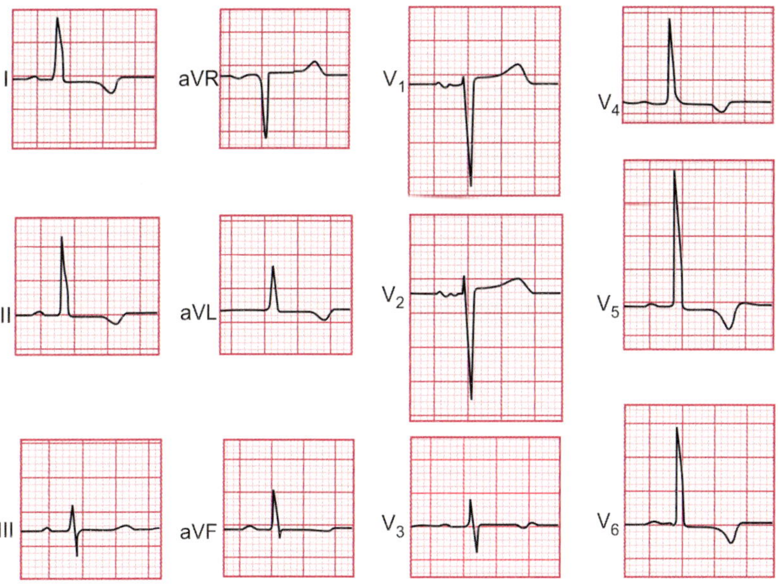


**Fig. 2.21**: Left ventricular hypertrophy

### *2.1.5.2. Right ventricular hypertrophy (RVH)*

1. The term infant: has physiological "normal" right ventricular hypertrophy .
2. • For pathological RVH, the mean QRS will move farther right and anteriorly.
   • In frontal plane QRS axes >190° for infant <1 week of age or 135° for infants > 1 month of age.
3. A "pure" R wave > 25 mm voltage, or a qR pattern in the right chest leads— This suggests  pathologic RVH in the newborn.
4. An upright or even "flat" T wave in $V_4R$ and $V_1$ in  a child between 1 week and 8 years of age is highly suggestive of RVH.
5. In an older adolescents, ECG criteria for RVH are:
   • Right axis deviation.
   • Increased R voltage in $V_1$ or S in $V_6$ and rsR' in $V_1$.
   • ST segment depression and a flipped T wave in $V_1$.

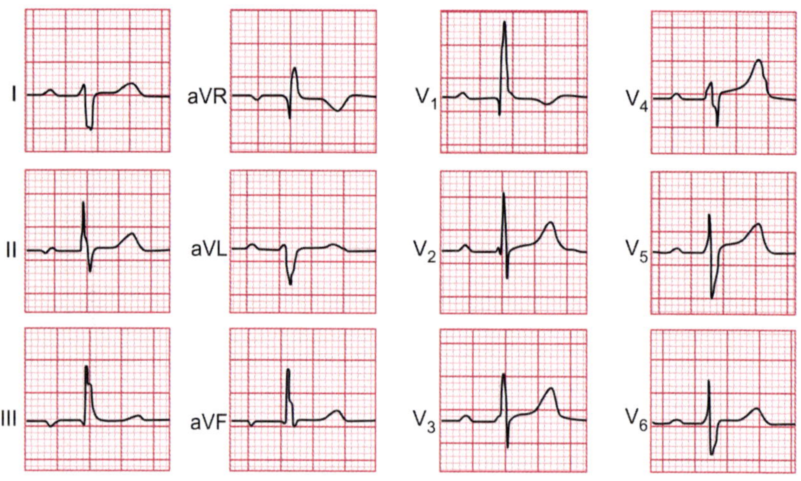

**Fig. 2.22**: Right ventricular hypertrophy

## 2.1. 6. Conduction disturbances

### 2.1.6.1. Atrioventricular (AV) blocks

### 1° AV block

- Prolongs the P–R interval more than normal for age and by > 200 ms (1 big square) beyond 16 years.

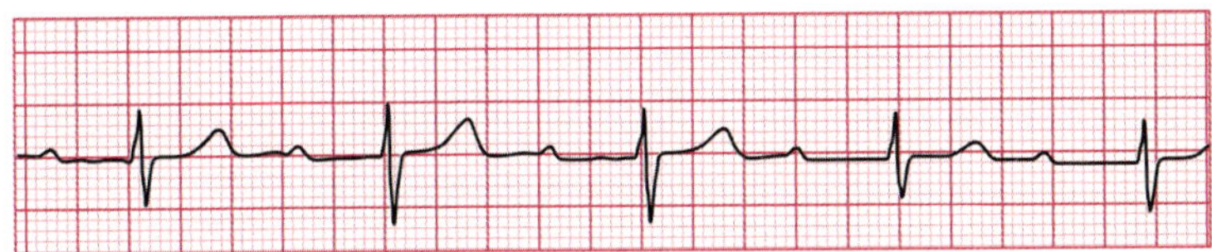

**Fig. 2.23**: First AV block

### 2° AV block results in 2 main patterns

**Mobitz I:**
- Wenckebach phenomenon involves progressive prolongation of the P–R interval until there is a drop in QRS (ventricular beat).
- Rarely requires treatment.

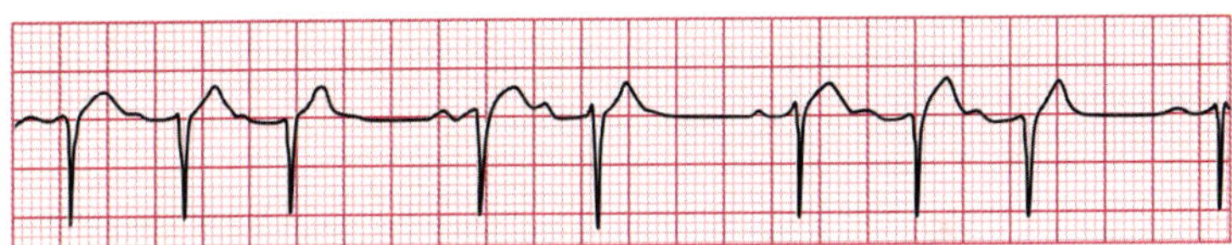

**Fig. 2.24**: Mobitz I, Second degree AV block

**Mobitz II:**
- Normal P–R interval, but, periodically, there is a drop in QRS
  - 2:1 AV block is 2 P waves for each QRS.
  - 3:1 AV block is 3 P waves for each QRS.
- Higher-grade heart block implies disease of the His-Purkinje conduction system.
- Often requires a pacemaker.

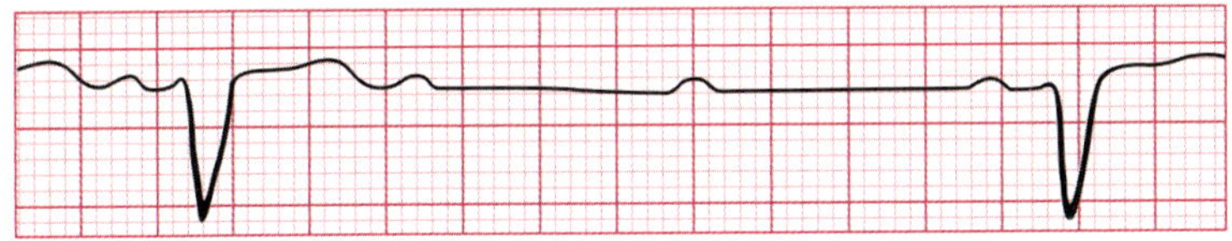

**Fig. 2.25**: Mobitz II, Second degree AV Block

## 3° AV block or complete heart block

- No atrial depolarizations are conducted through the AV node.
- If the QRS complex has a normal width (< 100 ms), there is a junctional ectopic pacemaker.
- Junctional escape rate is 40–60 bpm, whereas ventricular escape rate (which also would be a wider QRS) is 20–40 bpm.

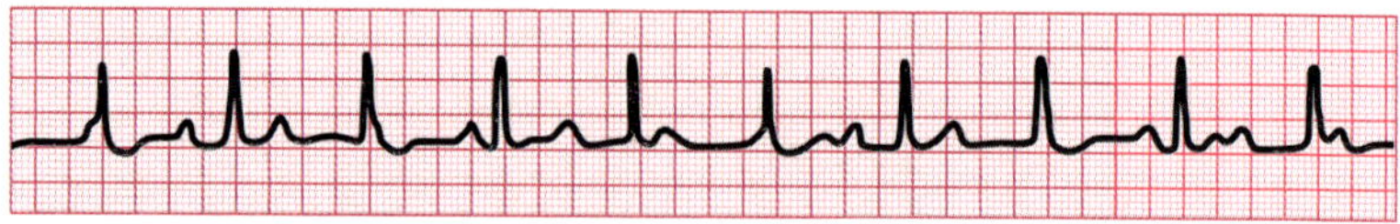

**Fig. 2.26**: Third degree AV block

### 2.1.6.2. Bundle branch block (BBB)

### 2.1.6.2. 1. LBBB

- It is rare in children.
- The QRS is prolonged, with a duration of 120–180 ms (3–4.5 small squares).
- An RR' (notched or slurred) in the lateral leads (I, aVL and $V_6$) and there is a corresponding SS' (also called QS ) in $V_1$.
- 50% of patients have a normal axis, 50% have LAD (–30° to –90°).

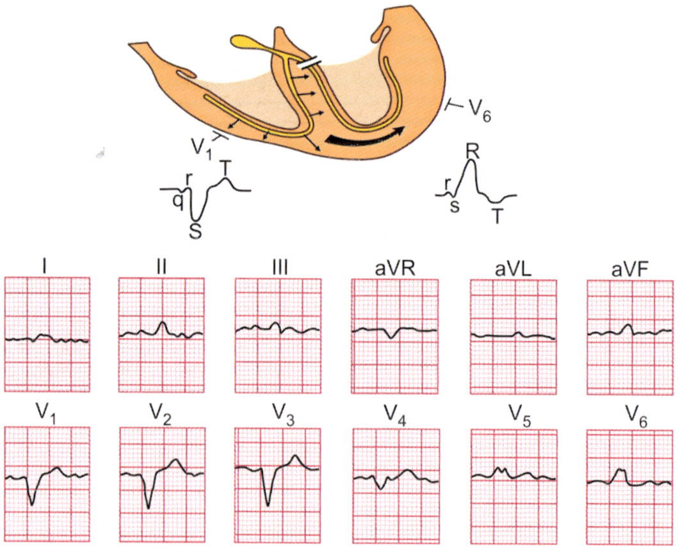


**Fig. 2.27**: Left bundle branch block

### 2.1.6.2. 2. RBBB

- More common in children, particularly after open heart surgery
- RR' or RSR' (rabbit ears) in $V_1$ and a wide S wave in $V_6$.

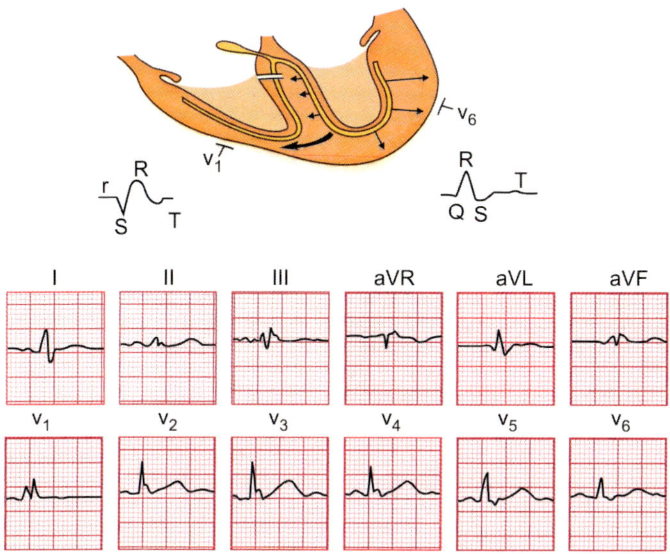

Fig. 2.28: Right bundle branch block

## 2.1.7. Areas of the ECG to be concentrated upon to study the events, e.g. MI

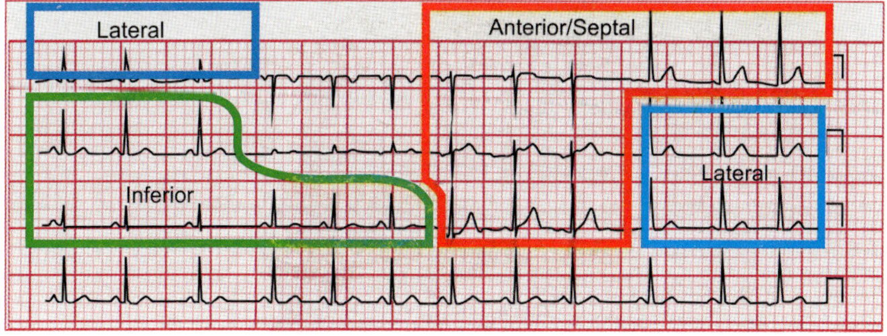


Fig. 2.29: Areas of ECG to evaluate the type of MI

| Position | Leads |
| --- | --- |
| Lateral | Look on lead I, $V_5$, $V_6$ |
| Inferior | Look on lead II, III, aVF |
| Anterior/septal | Look on $V_1$, $V_2$, $V_3$, $V_4$ |

## 2.2. Normal or Innocent Murmurs

| No | Murmur | Timing /Location /Quality | Usual age at diagnosis |
|---|---|---|---|
| 1 | Still's murmur/ vibratory murmur | Systolic ejection murmur | 3–6 years |
| | | LLSB or between LLSB and apex | |
| | | Grades I –III/VI | |
| | | Vibratory, musical quality | |
| | | Intensity decreases in upright position | |
| 2 | Venous hum | Continuous murmur | 3–6 years |
| | | Infraclavicular region (right >left) | |
| | | Grades I –III/VI | |
| | | Louder with patient in upright position | |
| | | Changes with compression of jugular vein or turning head | |
| 3 | Carotid bruit | Systolic ejection murmur | Any age |
| | | Neck, over carotid artery | |
| | | Grades I –III/VI | |
| 4 | Adolescent ejection murmur | Systolic ejection murmur | 8–14 years |
| | | LUSB | |
| | | Grades I –III/VI | |
| | | Usually softer in upright position | |
| | | Does not radiate to back | |
| 5 | Peripheral pulmonary stenosis | Systolic ejection murmur | 8–14 years |
| | | Axilla and back, LUSB/RUSB | |
| | | Grades I –II/VI | |
| | | Harsh, short, high-frequency | |

**N.B.** LLSB: Left lower sternal border, LUSB: Left upper sternal border, RUSB: Right upper sternal border

## 2.3. Cardiac Catheterization; Normal Heart

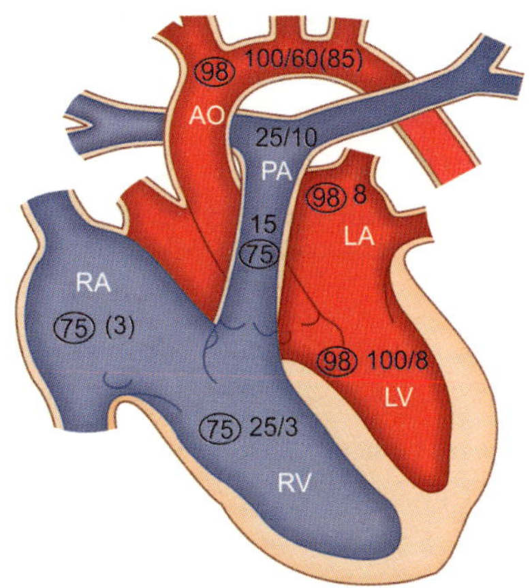


**Fig. 2.30**: Cardiac catheterization; normal heart
AO: Aorta; LA: Left atrium; LV: Left ventricle; PA: Pulmonary artery;
RA: Right atrium; RV: Right ventricle (circled values are oxygen saturations)

## 2.4. Congenital Heart Diseases

### 2.4.1. Genetic diseases and their associated cardiac abnormalities

#### 2.4.1.1. Single mutant gene syndrome

| | |
|---|---|
| Noonan syndrome | Pulmonary stenosis<br>Hypertrophic cardiomyopathy |
| Apert syndrome | VSD<br>Coarctation of aorta |
| Holt-Oram syndrome | ASD<br>VSD |
| Alagille syndrome | Pulmonary stenosis |
| Ellis-van Crevald syndrome | Single atrium |

#### 2.4.1.2. Chromosomal abnormalities

| | |
|---|---|
| Cri-du-chat syndrome | VSD |
| Turner syndrome (XO) | Bicuspid aortic valves<br>Coarctation of the aorta |
| Trisomy 21 (Down syndrome) | Endocardial cushion defect |
| Trisomy 13 (Patau syndrome) | VSD |
| Trisomy 18 (Edward syndrome) | VSD |

### 2.4.2. Left-to-right shunts occurring in "post-tricuspid" valve

1. **Aorta to pulmonary artery shunts:**
   - PDA.
   - Hemitruncus arteriosus.
   - Coronary-pulmonary fistula.
   - Left coronary artery anomalously originating from pulmonary artery.
2. **Aorta to right ventricle:**
   - Sinus of Valsalva fistula
   - Coronary arteiovenous fistula.
3. **Aorta to right atrium or vena cava:**
   - Systemic arteriovenous fistula
   - Sinus of Valsalva fistula.
4. **Left ventricle to right ventricle:**
   - VSD
   - Endocardial cushion defect.
5. **Left ventricle to right atrium:**
   - Left ventricle to right atrium connection
   - Endocardial cushion defect.

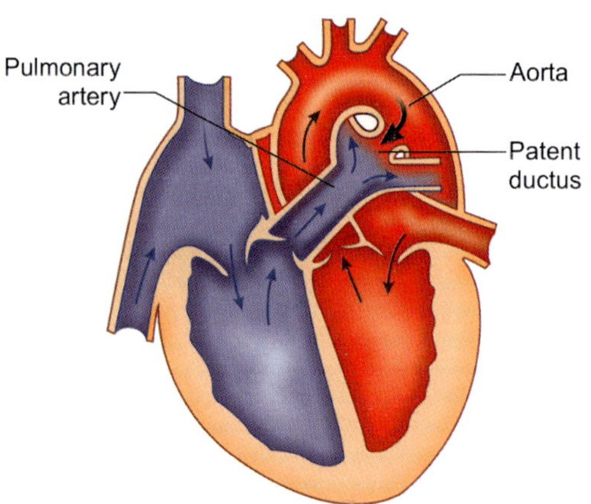


**Fig. 2.31**: Patent ductus arteriosus (PDA)

### *2.4.2.1. Patent ductus arteriosus (PDA)*

- The ductus arteriosus normally closes "functionally: within 10–15 hours after birth".
- Complete anatomic closure may not occur for 3 weeks.
- Premature infants (weighing <1.750 gm) have clinically apparent PDA ~ 40–70% of the time.

- Clinically, there is a continuous "rumbling" or "machinery-like" murmur and will usually increase in intensity in late systole.
- The best to be heard is below the left clavicle.
- There is a "collapsing" or "bounding" pulse.

### 2.4.2.2. Ventricular septal defect (VSD)

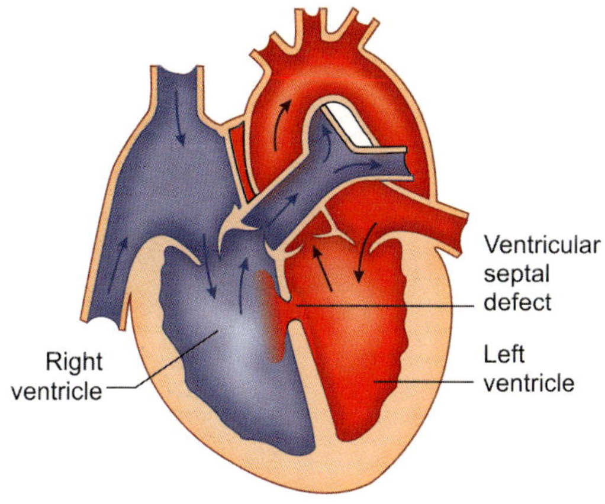


**Fig. 2.32**: Ventricular septal defect (VSD)

- VSDs are the most common congenital heart defects and make upto 25–30% of cases of congenital heart defects in term newborns.
- At birth, a majority of VSDs occur in the muscular septum but these usually close spontaneously ≤ 1 year of age.
- After 1 year, the majority of VSDs detected occur in the membranous septum.
- Clinically, there is "harsh" or high-pitched murmur.
- If the shunt is:
  - Small = only heard in early systole
  - Large = holosystolic.
- The best to be heard is at the lower left sternal border (LLSB), with maximal intensity near the subxiphoid area.
- Most symptoms will occur in term infants at 4–8 weeks of age and will consist of;
  - Volume overload
  - Heart failure.

### *2.4.2.3. Atrial septal defect (ASD)*

2.4.2.3.l. Ostium secundum defect

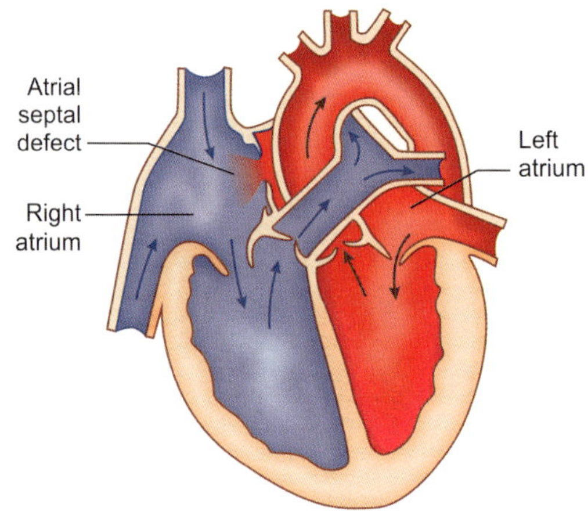


**Fig. 2.33**: Ostium secundum defect

- Ostium secundum defects are the most common form of ASD and are located in the midseptum.
- Older children with ASDs are usually asymptomatic.
- On physical examination:
  - $S_1$ is normal
  - $S_2$ is widely split without respiratory variation.
- The ASD itself does not usually produce a very loud murmur—The murmur is from increased flow across the right ventricular outflow tract and pulmonic valve.
- Chest X-ray can show:
  - The main pulmonary artery and right heart will be enlarged
  - Increased pulmonary blood flow.
- ECG will show:
  - RAD
  - RVH
  - Typical rsR or rsR' "Rabbit ears" in the right precordium
  - The S wave in the inferior leads and is usually notched.
- Pulmonary vascular disease with pulmonary hypertension can occur (~5%) but usually not until 20–30 years of age.
- Ostium secundum defects do not need endocarditis prophylaxis, nor does ostium primum.

### 2.4.2.3.2. Ostium primum defect

- Ostium primum defect is located in the lower portion of atrial septum. In the region of the mitral and tricuspid valves rings.
- Clinically, the left-right shunt results in right ventricular hypertrophy, with increased pulmonary blood flow
  So:
  – Right ventricular outflow murmur
  – tricuspid valve mid-diastolic murmur
  – Widely split $S_2$.
- ECG will show:
  – LAD
  – Right ventricular hypertrophy (RVH):
  * rsR' in the right precordium.
- LAD distinguishes the ostium primum defect from the ostium secundum defect.

### 2.4.2.3.3. Complete AV canal defect
### (AV septal defect, endocardial cushion defect)

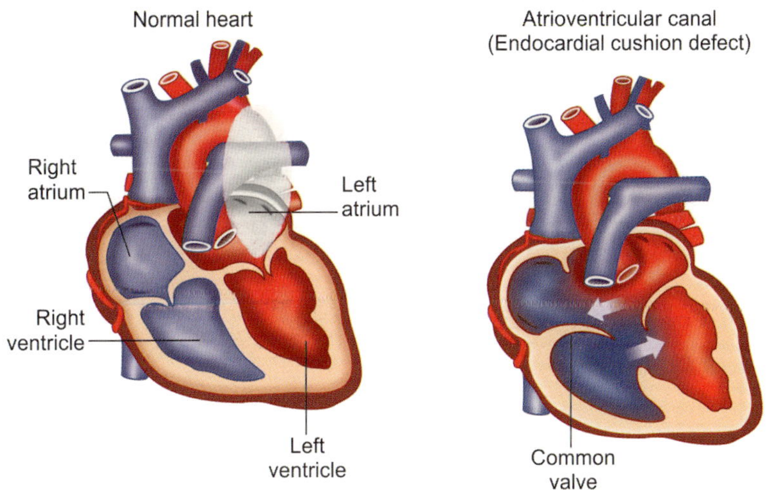


**Fig. 2.34**: Complete AV canal defect

- This involves failure of the "central" heart to develop, resulting in a large hole communication between the atria and ventricles, as well as malformation of the tricuspid and mitral valves.
- Clinically; a large left-to-right shunt and valve regurgitation → Cardiac volume overload and CHF.

- The infants most often present with heart failure by 2 months of age.
- This is the most common heart defect in Down syndrome (trisomy 21).
- Chest X-ray reveals:
  – Nonspecific, generalized cardiomegaly with increased pulmonary blood flow.
- ECG will usually show:
  – LAD
  – Prominent voltages with biventricular hypertrophy.
- Absence of these is very unusual for an AV canal defect.

Electrocardiogram of a 7-month-old male with a complete atrioventricular

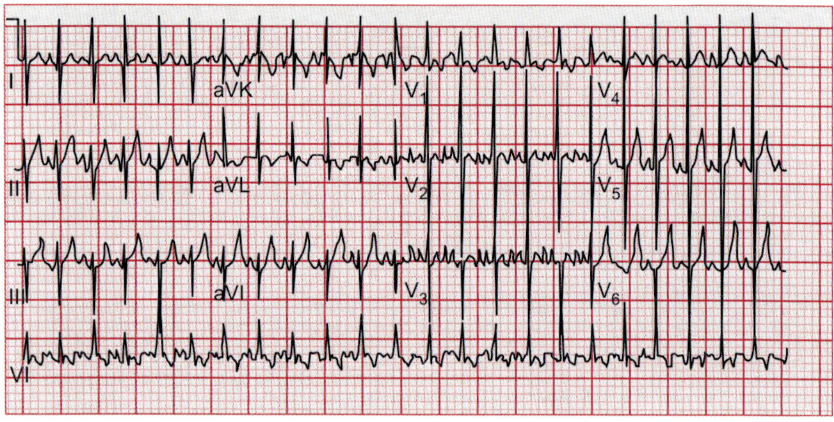

**Fig. 2.35**: ECG in complete AV canal defect

canal shows:
- Left axis deviation
- Biventricular hypertrophy are readily apparent
- Peaked p-waves in lead II suggests right atrial enlargement.

### 2.4.2.4. Coarctation of the aorta

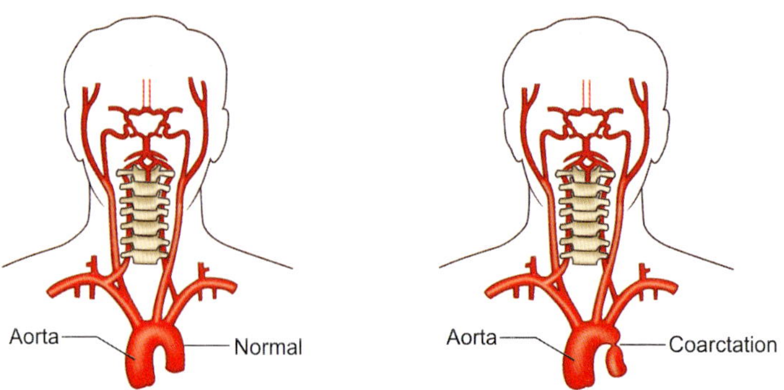


**Fig. 2.36**: Coarctation of the aorta

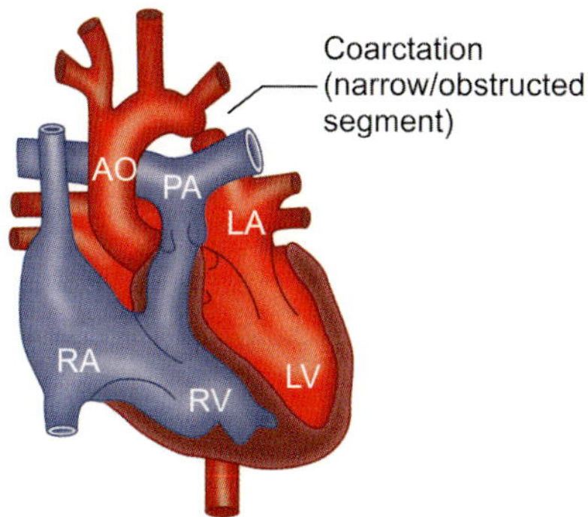



**Fig. 2.37**: Figure of coarctation of the aorta

- Coarctation develops from a defect in the vessel media, causing posterior infolding of the vessel.
  1. Clinically in infancy severe coarctation looks a like severe aortic stenosis, with "septic shock" appearance.
- Murmurs are not common, but if the ductus is patent, a continuous murmur along the left sternal border can be heard.
  2. Older kids may present with hypertension or murmur.
  3. Epistaxis, claudication-like symptoms in the lower extremities with exercise and headaches can happen but are uncommon.
- Stroke is rare <7years of age, but if it occurs, it is likely associated with a rupture berry aneurysm.
- Diagnosis is from pulses and blood pressure—Not from murmurs.
- Pulses in the upper extremities are strong with associated hypertension, while the femoral pulses are absent or weak.

**Chest X-ray shows:**
- The area of dilatation below the coarctation and the dilated aortic segment just above the coarctation of aortic arch → "3" sign if you look down the left upper border of the aortic arch and descending aorta.
- Rib notching is classic, but may not develop for 5–6 years occurs
  – At the lower margins of the ribs, at about the middle third
  – In >50% of affected older children.

## 2.4.3. Right-to-left shunts

### 2.4.3.1. Tetralogy of Fallot (TOF)

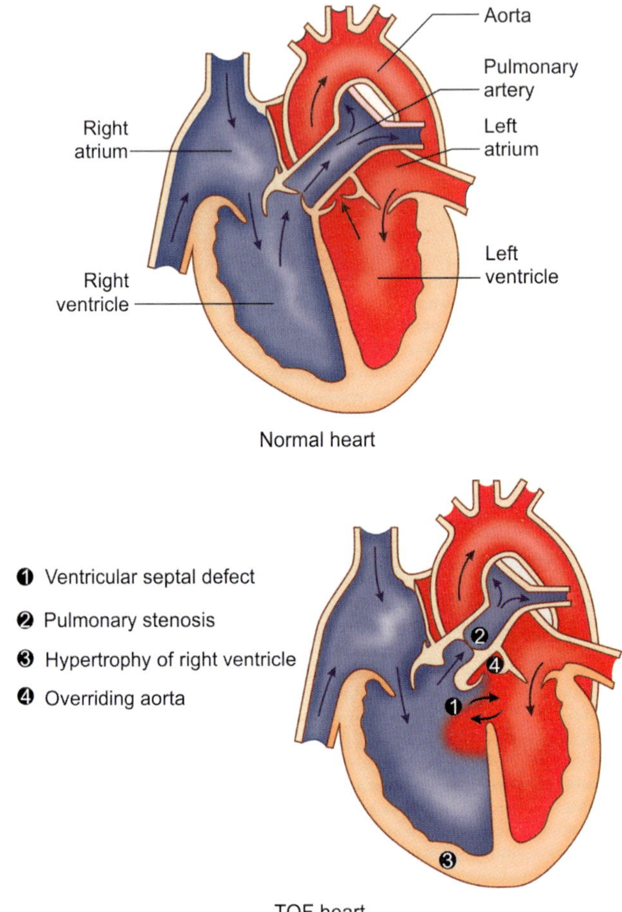



**Fig. 2.38**: TOF vs. normal heart

- The most common cyanotic heart lesion in children with congenital heart disease who have survived untreated beyond infancy.
- It makes upto 7–10% of congenital defects.

Four things make up the tetralogy (see picture above)

1. RV outflow tract obstruction (subpulmonary valve stenosis)
2. VSD (malalignment)
3. Overriding aorta (dextropositioning)
4. RVH.

The child with TOF is at risk for:

1. Brain abscess
2. Cerebral thrombosis with hemiplegia
3. Infective endocarditis
   - Clinically, squatting  after exercise can occur
   - Systolic murmur best heard at the middle or left lower sternal border
   - Chest X-ray classically shows:
     – The "boot-shaped" heart or "Coeur en sabot"
     – 25–30% have a right aortic arch.
   - ECG will show:
     – RAD and RVH.

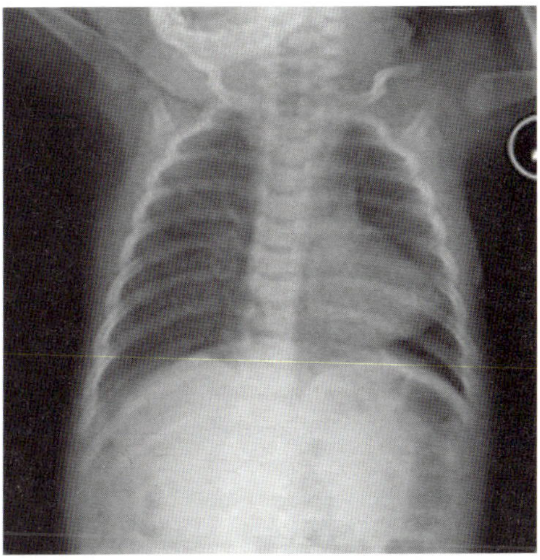

**Fig. 2.39**: X-ray of child with TOF

## 2.4.3.2. Transposition of great arteries (TGA)

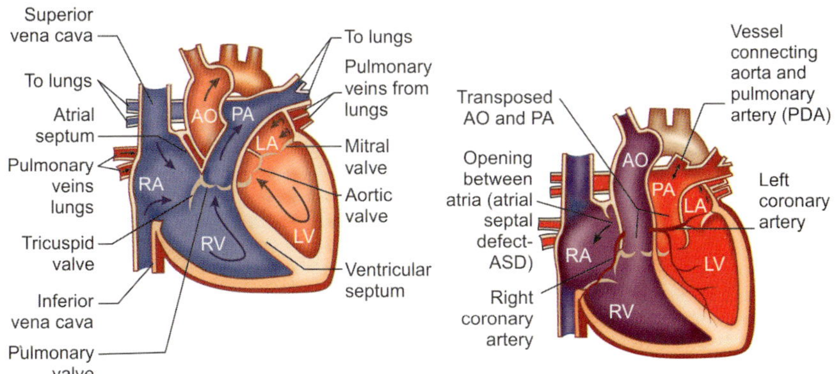


**Fig. 2.40**: Transposition of great arteries vs. normal heart

- TGA is the most common cardiac cause of cyanosis in the newborn during the first few days of life.
  NB. TOF is the most common for all ages together.
- It comprises 4–6% of congenital defects.
- The only initial presenting signs/symptoms in an otherwise healthy appearing baby may be severe cyanosis in an infant with TGA without a VSD.

*Clinically*:
- Single, loud second sound will be heard.
- 2–3/6, nonspecific, systolic ejection murmur at the middle left sternal border.
- If an associated VSD is present in an infant, CHF and modest Cyanosis will develop by 3–4 weeks of age.
- These infants usually have tachypnea and dyspnea.
- Chest X-ray can be:
  – Normal or
  – Classic finding: Egg-shaped or oval-shaped heart with a narrow mediastinum and small thymus. It is seen in only ~33% of affected infants.
- ECG may be helpful after ~5 days, with a persistently positive T wave in the right precordium.

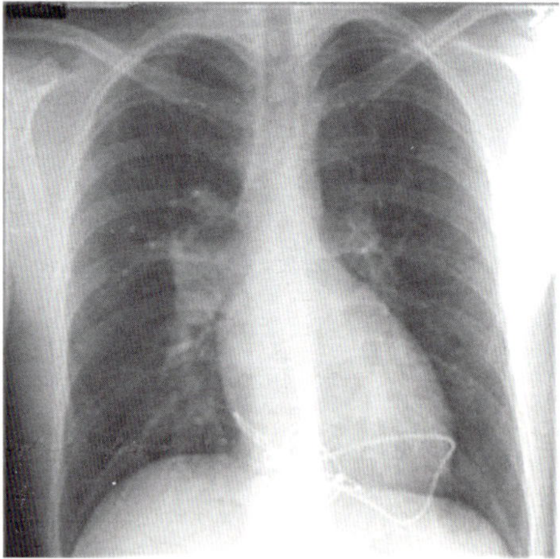

**Fig. 2.41**: X-ray in a child with transposition of great arteries

## Bibliography


1. http://www.congenitalcardiologytoday.com/
2. http://www.hopkinsmedicine.org/heart_vascular_institute/conditions_treatments/conditions/pediatric_congenital_heart_disease.html.
3. http://www.mayoclinic.org

# Dentistry

## 3.1. The Times of Eruption of the Primary and Permanent Teeth

### 3.1.1. Primary dentition

**Primary Dentition**

| Maxillary | | |
|---|---|---|
| **Tooth** | **Range** | |
| Central incisor | 4 months | 7½ months |
| Lateral incisor | 5 months | 8 months |
| Canine | 9 months | 16–20 months |
| First molar | 6 months | 12–16 months |
| Second molar | 10–12 months | 20–30 months |
| **Mandibular** | | |
| **Tooth** | **Range** | |
| Central incisor | 4 months | 6½ months |
| Lateral incisor | 4¼ months | 7 months |
| Canine | 9 months | 16–20 months |
| First molar | 6 months | 12–16 months |
| Second molar | 10–12 months | 20–30 months |

### 3.1.2. Permanent dentition

**Permanent Dentition**

| Maxillary | | |
|---|---|---|
| **Tooth** | **Range** | |
| Central incisor | 4–5 years | 7–8 years |
| Lateral incisor | 4–5 years | 8–9 years |
| Canine | 6–7 years | 11–12 years |

*Contd...*

*Contd...*

| Tooth | Range | |
|---|---|---|
| First premolar | 5–6 years | 10–11 years |
| Second premolar | 6–7 years | 10–12 years |
| First molar | 2½–3 years | 6–7 years |
| Second molar | 7–8 years | 12–13 years |
| Third molar | 12–16 years | 17–21 years |
| **Mandibular** | | |
| **Tooth** | **Range** | |
| Central incisor | 4–5 years | 6–7 years |
| Lateral incisor | 4–5 years | 7–8 years |
| Canine | 6–7 years | 9–10 years |
| First premolar | 5–6 years | 10–12 years |
| Second premolar | 6–7 years | 11–12 years |
| First molar | 2½–3 years | 6–7 years |
| Second molar | 7–8 years | 11–13 years |
| Third molar | 12–16 years | 17–21 years |

## 3.2. Angle Classification of Occlusion

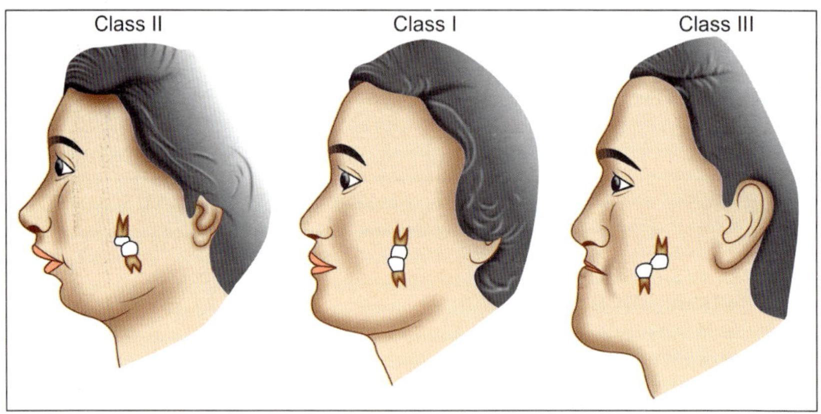


**Fig. 3.1**: Angle classification of occlusion

The typical correspondence between the facial-jaw profile and molar relationship is shown

## 3.3. Traumatic Oral Injury

Traumatic oral injuries may be categorized into three groups:
1. Injuries to teeth.
2. Injuries to soft tissue (contusions, abrasions, lacerations, punctures, avulsions and burns).
3. Injuries to jaw (mandibular or maxillary fractures or both).

### 3.3.1. Injuries to teeth

- Approximately 10% of children between 18 months and 18 years of age will sustain significant tooth trauma.
- The three age groups with greatest predilection are:
  1. Toddlers (1–3 years), usually due to:
     i. Falls
     ii. Child abuse.
  2. School-aged (7–10 years), usually from:
     i. Bicycle
     ii. Playground accidents.
  3. Adolescents (16–18 years), often the result of:
     i. Fights
     ii. Athletic injuries
     iii. Automobile accidents.

### *3.3.1.1. Tooth fractures*

I. Tooth fractures may involve:
   1. Enamel
   2. Dentin
   3. Pulp.
II. They may occur in:
   1. The crown
   2. The root of a tooth.

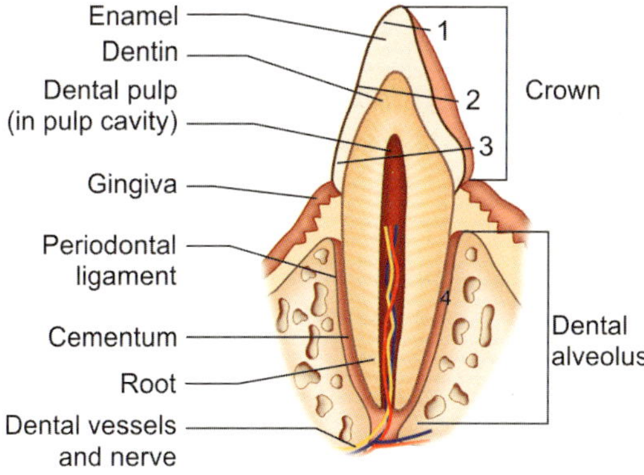


**Fig. 3.2**: Areas of tooth fractures

### 3.4. Discolored Teeth

1. Neonatal hyperbilirubinemia (blue to black discoloration of the primary teeth).
2. Porphyria (red-brown discoloration).
3. Tetracyclines (brown-yellow discoloration and hypoplasia of the enamel).

### 3.5. Conditions Associated with Natal Teeth

1. Cleft palate
2. Pierre Robin syndrome
3. Ellis-van Creveld syndrome
4. Hallermann-Streiff syndrome
5. Pachyonychia congenita
6. Other anomalies.

### 3.6. Systemic Problems that Cause Aggressive Periodontitis in Children

1. Neutropenia
2. Leukocyte adhesion or migration defects
3. Hypophosphatasia
4. Papillon-Lefèvre syndrome
5. Leukemia
6. Histiocytosis X.

### 3.7. Differential Diagnosis of Oral Ulceration

| Common | |
| --- | --- |
| **Condition** | **Comment** |
| Aphthous (canker sore) | Painful and circumscribed lesions; recurrences |
| Traumatic | Accidents, chronic cheek biter, or after dental local anesthesia |
| Hand, foot and mouth disease | Painful; lesions on tongue, anterior oral cavity, hands and feet |
| Herpangina | Painful; lesions confined to soft palate and oropharynx |
| Herpetic gingivostomatitis | Vesicles on mucocutaneous borders; painful and febrile |
| Recurrent herpes labialis | Vesicles on lips; painful |
| Chemical burns | Alkali, acid, aspirin; painful |
| Heat burns | Hot food and electrical |

| Uncommon | |
| --- | --- |
| **Condition** | **Comment** |
| Neutrophil defects | Agranulocytosis, leukemia, cyclic neutropenia; painful |
| Systemic lupus erythematosus | Recurrent, may be painless |
| Behçet's syndrome | Resembles aphthous lesions; associated with genital ulcers and uveitis |
| Necrotizing ulcerative gingivostomatitis | Vincent stomatitis; painful |
| Syphilis | Chancre or gumma; painless |
| Oral Crohn disease | Aphthous-like; painful |
| Histoplasmosis | Lingual |

## 3.8. Bilateral Enlargement of the Submaxillary Glands

Bilateral enlargement of the submaxillary glands can occur in:
1. AIDS
2. Cystic fibrosis
3. Epstein-Barr virus infection
4. Malnutrition.

## 3.9. Benign Salivary Gland Hypertrophy

Benign salivary gland hypertrophy has been associated with:
1. Endocrinopathies
2. Thyroid disease
3. Diabetes
4. Disorders of the pituitary-adrenal axis.

## 3.10. Xerostomia

| Xerostomia (dry mouth) may be associated with: | |
| --- | --- |
| 1. Fever | 5. Mikulicz disease (leukemia infiltrates) |
| 2. Dehydration | 6. Sjögren syndrome |
| 3. Anticholinergic drugs | 7. Tumoricidal doses of radiation when the salivary glands are within the field |
| 4. Chronic graft versus host disease | |

## Bibliography


1. http://ejo.oxfordjournals.org/content/22/2/169.full.pdf
2. http://my.clevelandclinic.org/services/dental_care/hic_teeth_eruption_timetable.aspx
3. http://www.rch.org.au/clinicalguide/guideline_index/Dental_Injuries/

# Dermatology

## 4.1. Skin Lesions

### 4.1.1. Primary skin lesions

Primary lesions are classified as:
1. Macules
2. Papules
3. Patches
4. Plaques
5. Nodules
6. Tumors
7. Vesicles
8. Bullae
9. Pustules
10. Wheals
11. Cysts.

### *4.1.1.1. Definition of primary skin lesions*

1. Macule represents an alteration in skin color but cannot be felt.
2. Patch when the macule is >1 cm, the term is used.
3. Papules are palpable solid lesions <1 cm.
4. Plaques are aggregations of papules.
5. Nodules are larger in diameter and deeper in the skin than papules
6. Tumors are solid raised mass having a diameter larger than 1 cm with the dimension of depth, usually larger than nodules and vary considerably in mobility and consistency.
7. Vesicles are raised, fluid-filled lesions <0.5 cm in diameter.
8. Bullae are larger vesicles.
9. Pustules contain purulent material.
10. Wheals are flat-topped, palpable lesions of variable size, duration, and configuration that represent dermal collections of edema fluid.
11. Cysts are circumscribed, thick-walled lesions; they are covered by a normal epidermis and contain fluid or semisolid material.

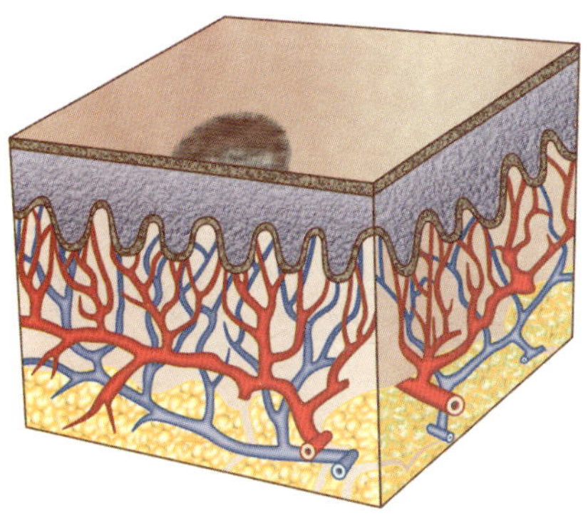

**A. Macule**
(e.g. freckles and moles)

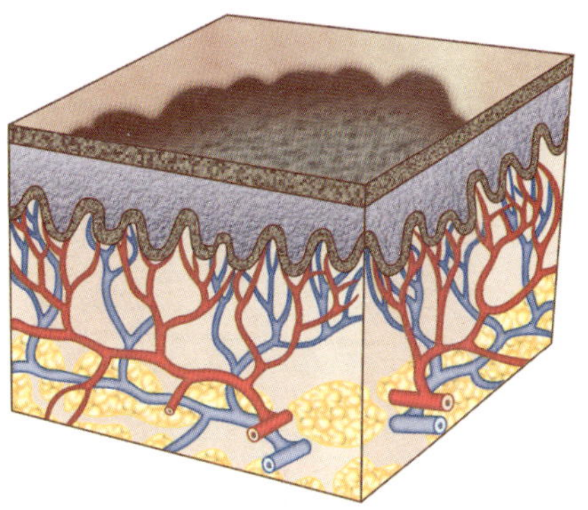

**B. Patch**
(e.g. vitiligo and café au lait spots)

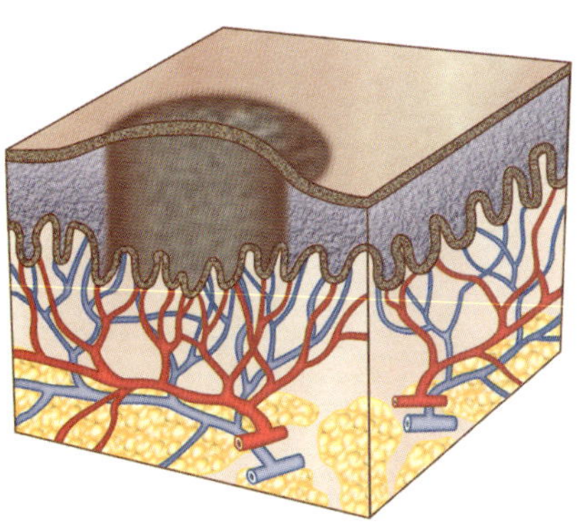

**C. Papule**
(e.g. nevus and wart)

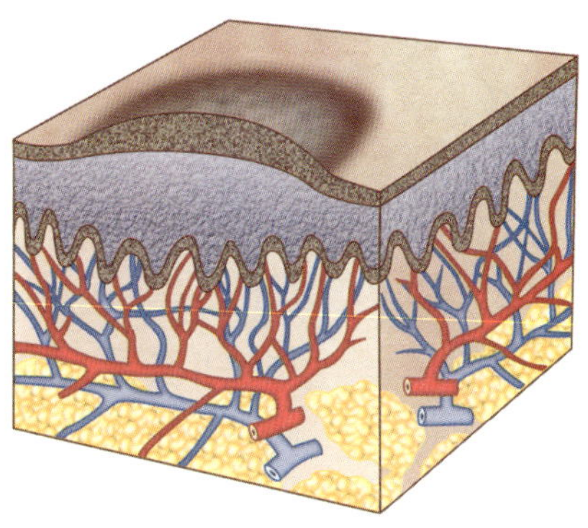

**D. Plaque**
(e.g. psoriasis and seborrheic keratosis)

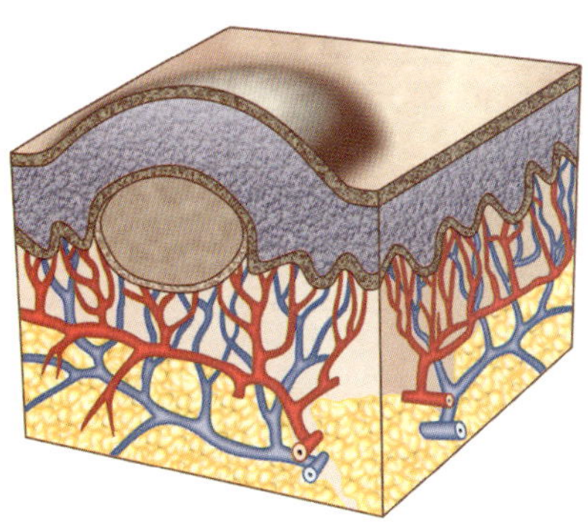

**E. Nodule**
(e.g. erythema nodosum)

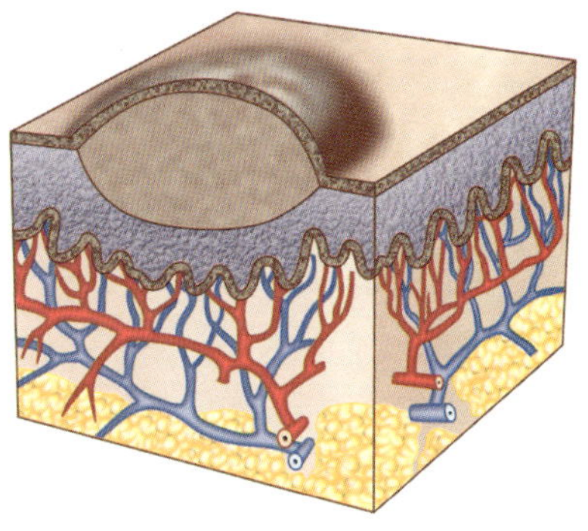

**F. Tumor**
(e.g. neoplasms)

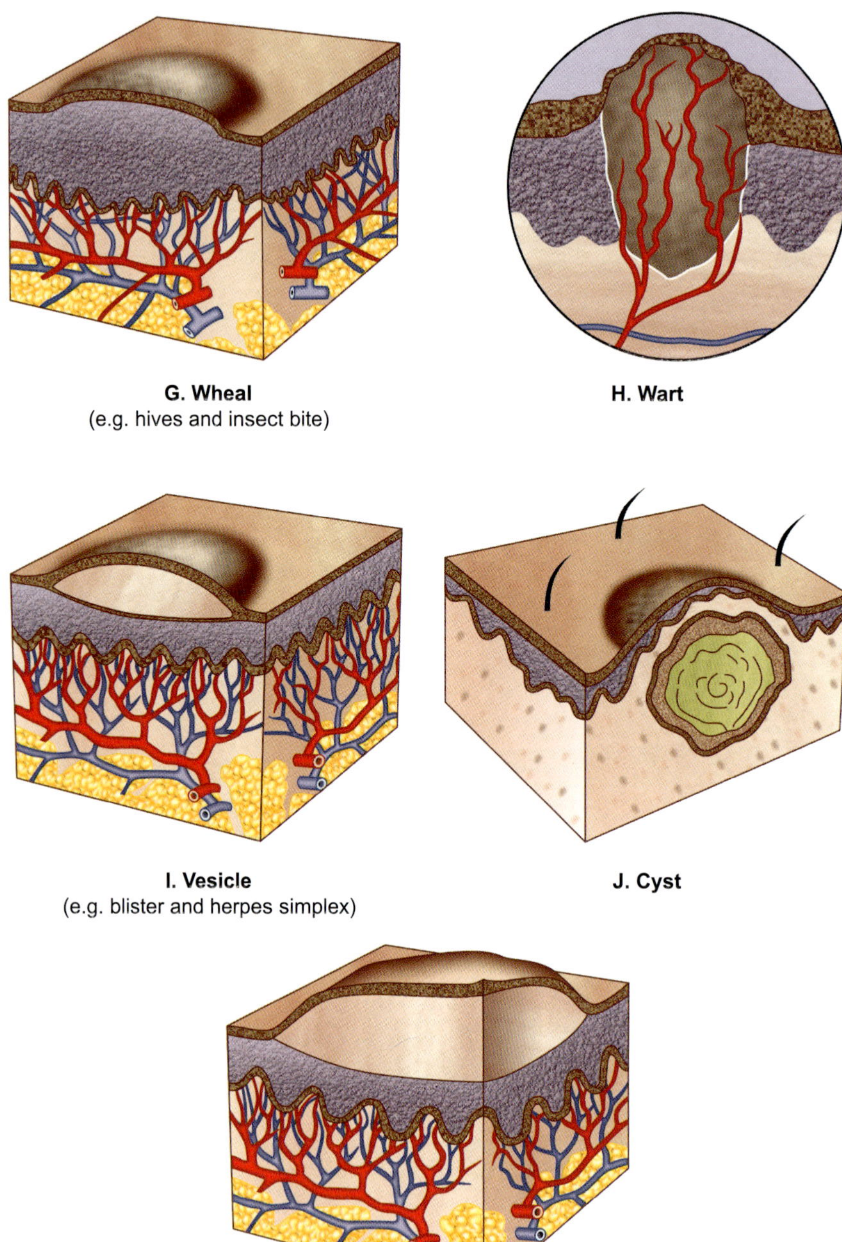



**Figs 4.1A to K**: Primary skin lesions

## 4.1.2. Secondary skin lesions

Secondary lesions include
1.  Scales
2.  Ulcers
3.  Erosions
4.  Excoriations
5.  Fissures
6.  Crusts
7.  Scars
8.  Lichenification.

### *4.1.2.1. Definition of secondary skin lesions*

- **Scales** consist of compressed layers of stratum corneum cells that are retained on the skin surface.
- **Erosions** involve focal loss of the epidermis, and they heal without scarring.
- **Ulcers** extend into the dermis and tend to heal with scarring.
- **Excoriations** is ulcerated lesions inflicted by scratching are often linear or angular in configuration.
- **Fissures** are caused by splitting or cracking; they usually occur in diseased skin.
- **Crusts** consist of matted, retained accumulations of blood, serum, pus, and epithelial debris on the surface of a weeping lesion.
- **Scars** are end-stage lesions that can be thin, depressed and atrophic, raised and hypertrophic, or flat and pliable; they are composed of fibrous connective tissue.
- **Lichenification** is a thickening of skin with accentuation of normal skin lines that is caused by chronic irritation (rubbing and scratching) or inflammation.

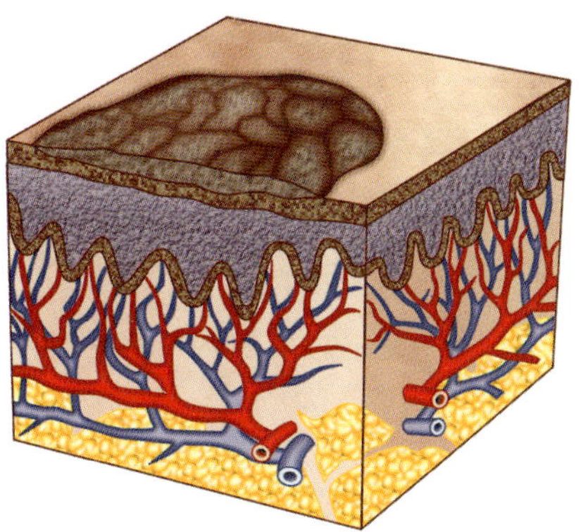

**A. Scale**
(e.g. dandruff and psoriasis)

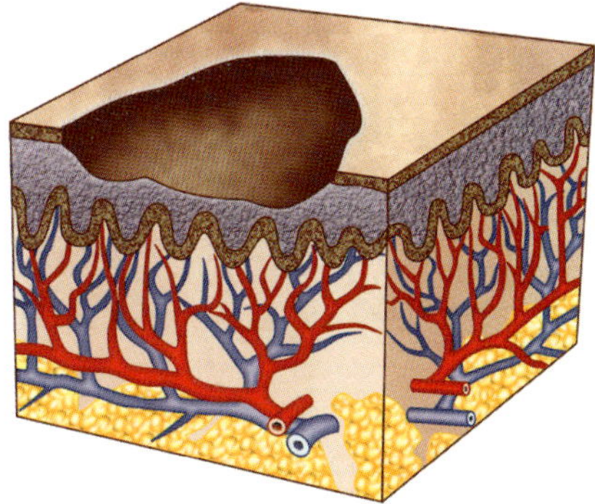

**B. Erosion**
(e.g. rupture of a vesicle)

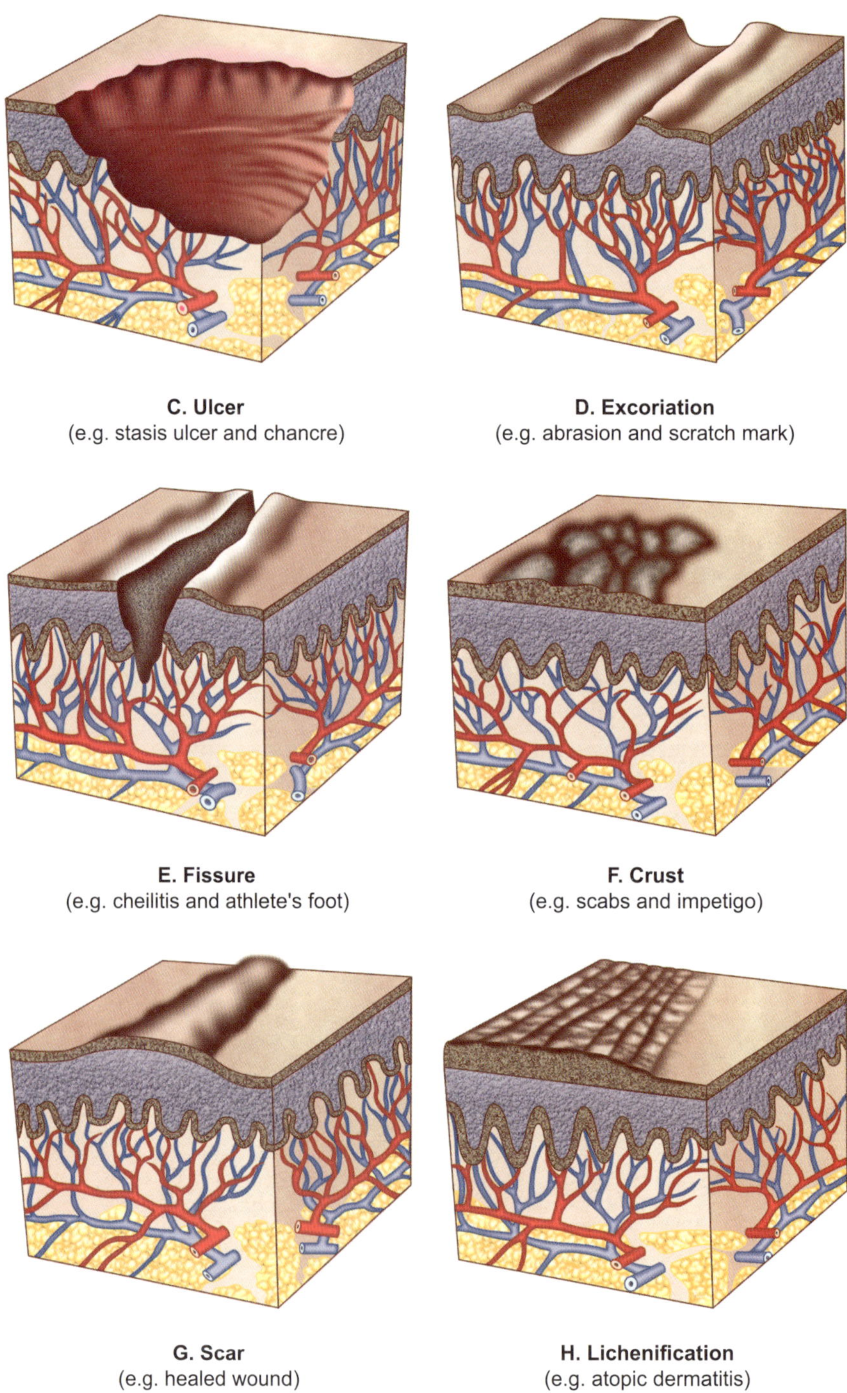

**C. Ulcer**
(e.g. stasis ulcer and chancre)

**D. Excoriation**
(e.g. abrasion and scratch mark)

**E. Fissure**
(e.g. cheilitis and athlete's foot)

**F. Crust**
(e.g. scabs and impetigo)

**G. Scar**
(e.g. healed wound)

**H. Lichenification**
(e.g. atopic dermatitis)

**Figs 4.2A to H**: Secondary skin lesions

## 4.2. Nonpathological Neonatal Skin Lesions

1. Sebaceous hyperplasia
2. Milia
3. Cutis marmoráta
4. Harlequin color change
5. Salmon patch (nevus simplex)
6. Mongolian spots
7. Erythema toxicum
8. Transient neonatal pustular melanosis.

1. **Sebaceous hyperplasia:**
   - Minute, profuse, yellow-white papules are frequently found on the forehead, nose, upper lip and cheeks of a term infant.
   - They represent hyperplastic sebaceous glands.

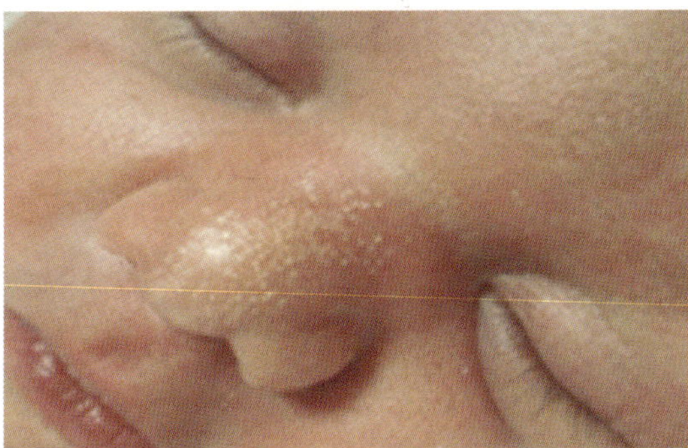

**Fig. 4.3**: Sebaceous hyperplasia

2. **Milia:** These are superficial epidermal inclusion cysts that contain laminated kerati-nized material.

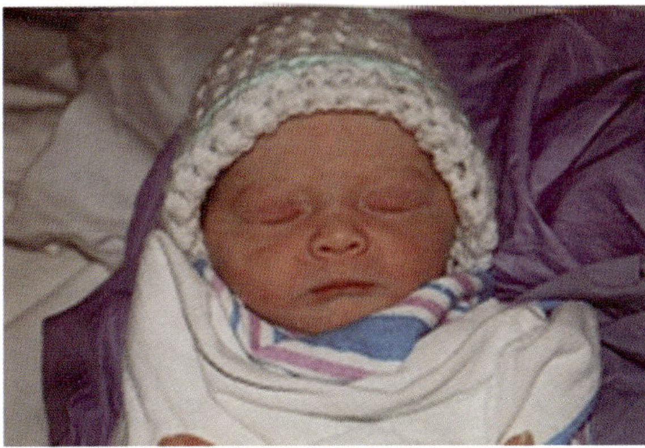

**Fig. 4.4**: Milia

3. **Cutis marmoráta:**
   - An evanescent, lacy, reticulated red and/or blue cutaneous vascular pattern appears over most of the body surface.
   - When a newborn infant is exposed to low environmental temperatures.
4. **Harlequin color change:**

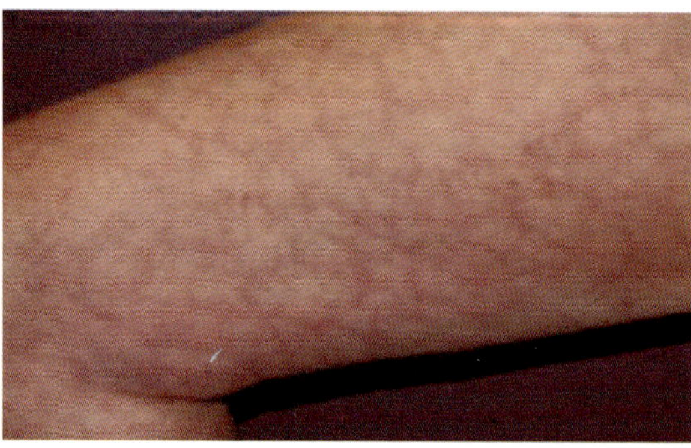

Fig. 4.5: Cutis marmorata

   - Occurs in the immediate newborn period and is most common in low birth weight (LBW) infants.
   - It probably reflects an imbalance in the autonomic vascular regulatory mechanism.
   - The color change lasts only for a few minutes and occasionally affects only a portion of the trunk or face.
   - Changing the infant's position may reverse the pattern.
5. **Salmon patch (nevus simplex):**

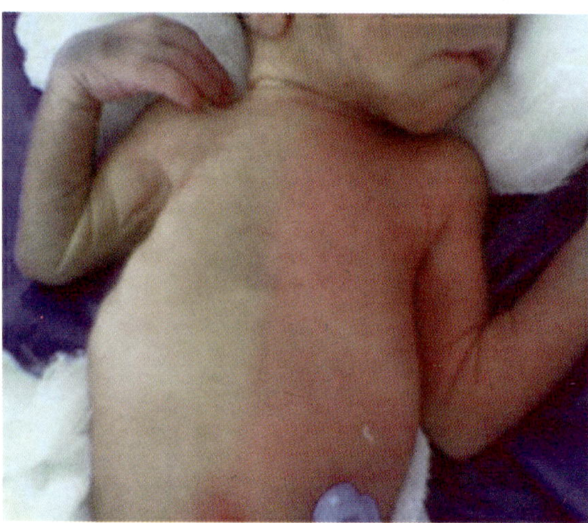

Fig. 4.6: Harlequin color change

- These are small, pale pink, ill-defined, vascular macules that occur most commonly on the glabella, eyelids, upper lip, and  nuchal area of 30–40% of normal newborn infants.
- Represent localized vascular ectasia.
- Persist for several months and may become more visible during crying or changes in environmental temperature.

6. **Mongolian spots:**

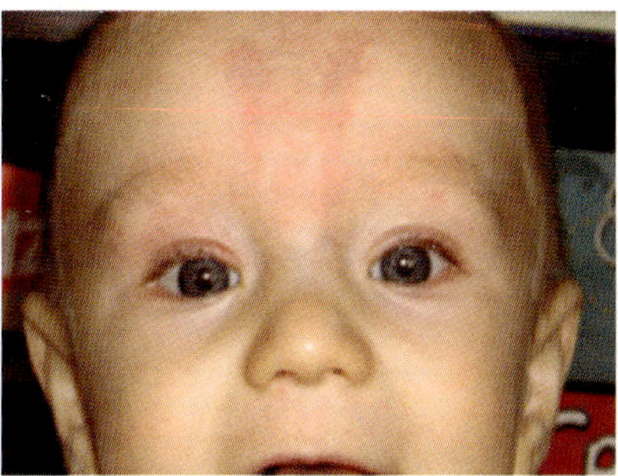

**Fig. 4.7**: Salmon patch

- Blue or slate-gray macular lesions, have variably defined margins.
- They occur most commonly in the presacral area but may be found over the posterior thighs, legs, back and shoulders.
- More than 80% of black, Asian and East Indian infants have these lesions, whereas the incidence in white infants is <10%.
- The peculiar hue of these macules is due to the dermal location of melanin-containing melanocytes that are presumably arrested in their migration from neural crest to epidermis.

7. **Erythema toxicum:**

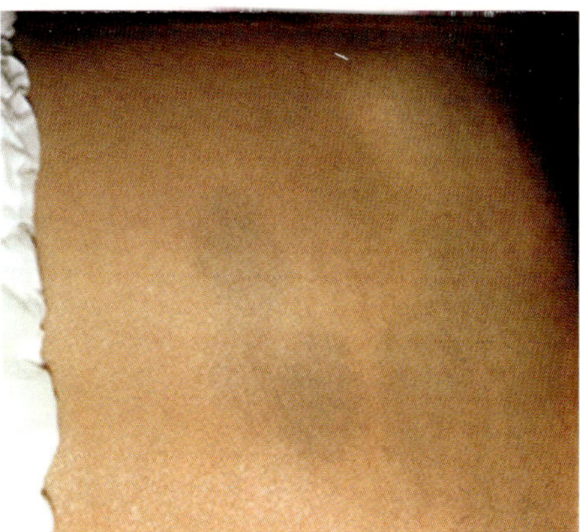

**Fig. 4.8**: Mongolian spots

- A benign, self-limited and evanescent eruption.
- Occurs in ≈ 50% of full-term infants; preterm infants are affected less commonly.
- The lesions are firm, yellow-white, 1–2 mm papules or pustules with a surrounding erythematous flare.
- Peak incidence occurs on the 2nd day of life.
- The eosinophils can be demonstrated in Wright-stained smears of the intralesional contents.

8. **Transient neonatal pustular melanosis:**

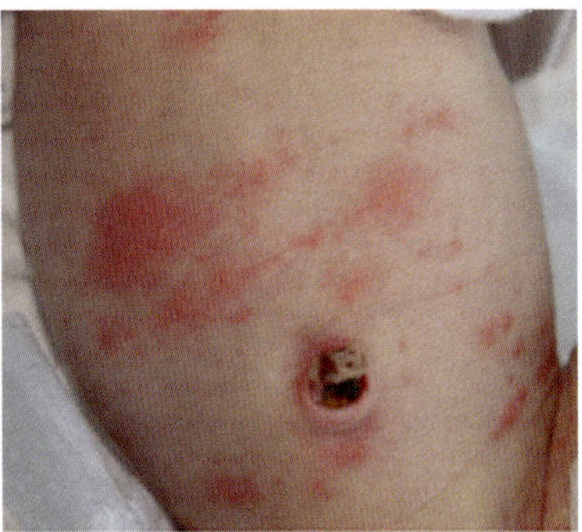

**Fig. 4.9**: Erythema toxicum

- It is more common among black than among white infants  .
- It is a transient, benign and self-limited dermatosis of unknown cause.
- It is characterized by 3 types of lesions:
  - Evanescent superficial pustules.
  - Ruptured pustules with a collarette of fine scale, at times with a central hyperpigmented macule.
  - Hyperpigmented macules.

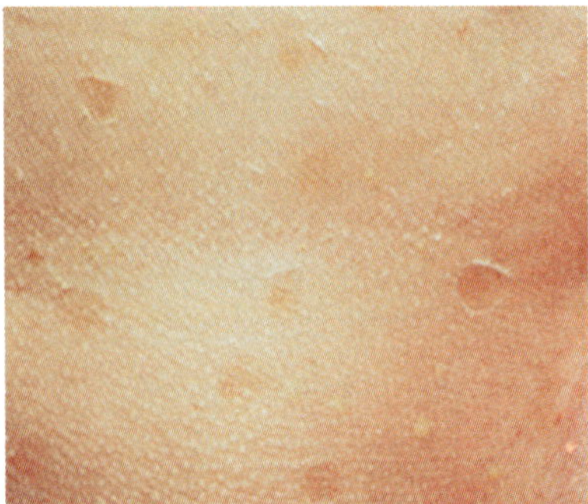

**Fig. 4.10**: Transient neonatal pustular melanosis

## 4.3. Disorders with Café-au-lait Spots

- Neurofibromatosis
- McCune-Albright syndrome
- Russell-Silver syndrome
- Ataxia telangiectasia
- Fanconi anemia
- Tuberous sclerosis
- Bloom syndrome
- Basal cell nevus syndrome
- Gaucher disease
- Chédiak-Higashi syndrome
- Hunter syndrome
- Maffucci syndrome
- Multiple mucosal neuroma syndrome
- Watson syndrome.

## Bibliography


1. http://dermnetnz.org/vascular/cutis-marmorata.html
2. http://www.derm-hokudai.jp/shimizu-dermatology/pdf/04-02.pdf
3. http://www.dermrounds.com/photo
4. http://www.pediatriconcall.com/fordoctor/imagegallery
5. http://www.pediatrics.wisc.edu/education/derm/text.htm
6. http://www.webmd.com/skin-problems-and-treatments/picture-of-erythema-toxicum-neonatorum
7. http://www.webmd.com/skin-problems-and-treatments/picture-of-mongolian-spots
8. http://www.webmd.com/skin-problems-and-treatments/picture-of-transient-neonatal-pustular-melanosis.
9. Stephan MR, Kirby MB, Blackwell KM. Common newborn Dermatologic conditions. Clinics in Family Practice 5(3). September 2003.

# Endocrinology

## 5.1. Relationship between Average Blood Glucose Level (mmol/L) and 'Glycosylated Hemoglobin' (HbA1c)

1. 'Glycosylated hemoglobin' (HbA1c) is a form of hemoglobin that is measured primarily to identify the average plasma glucose concentration over prolonged periods of time usually 8–12 weeks.
2. (HbA1c) levels by coincidence nearly equate to glucose levels.
3. A normal nondiabetic HbA1c is 3.5–5.5%.
4. In diabetes about 6.5% is good.

| HbA1c% | Average blood glucose level mmol/L |
|---|---|
| 13 | 18 |
| 12 | 17 |
| 11 | 15 |
| 10 | 13 |
| 9 | 12 |
| 8 | 10 |
| 7 | 8 |
| 6 | 7 |
| 5 | 5 |

## 5.2. Drugs and Conditions that Affect Thyroid Function Tests

| Increased TBG | Decreased TBG | Blocks peripheral conversion of $T_4$–$T_3$ | Blocks thyroid release of $T_4$ and $T_3$ |
|---|---|---|---|
| • Estrogen:<br>  – Supplements<br>  – Contraceptives<br>  – Pregnancy | • Androgens<br>• Glucocorticoids | • Propranolol<br>• Glucocorticoids | • Lithium |
| • Tamoxifen<br>• Clofibrate<br>• Narcotics | • Nephrotic syndrome | • Propylthiouracil | • Iodine |

*Contd...*

*Contd...*

| Increased TBG | Decreased TBG | Blocks peripheral conversion of $T_4$–$T_3$ | Blocks thyroid release of $T_4$ and $T_3$ |
|---|---|---|---|
| • Hepatitis<br>• Biliary cirrhosis | • Genetics<br>• Familial | • Amiodarone | |

## 5.3. Overview of a Thyroid Function Workup

| 1st test | 2nd test | | 3rd test |
|---|---|---|---|
| sTSH | $FT_4I$, $FT_4E$, $FT_4$ | Clinical status | |
| High | Low | Primary hypothyroidism | N/A |
| | Normal | Incipient/subclinical hypothyroidism | TRH to confirm |
| | High | Pituitary hyperthyroidism | N/A |
| Low | High | Thyrotoxicosis | RAIU |
| | Normal | Incipient /subclinical hyperthyroidism | TRH to confirm |
| | Low | Pituitary hypothyroidism | N/A |

N.B.N/A: Nonapplicable, RAIU: Radioiodine uptake

## 5.4. Symmetrical Goiter

| Clinically | $FT_4$ | TSH | ATA | Anti TPO | TSI | Imaging |
|---|---|---|---|---|---|---|
| Hypo | Yes | Yes | Yes | Yes | No | No |
| Hyper | Yes | Yes | Yes | Yes | Yes | No |
| Euthyroid | Yes | Yes | Yes | Yes | No | No |
| Imaging usually is not necessary for goiter but occasionally may be helpful for hyperthyroidism with goiter | | | | | | |

ATA: Antithyroid antibodies; Anti TPO: Antithyroid peroxidase antibodies; TSI: Thyroid stimulating immunoglobulin

## 5.5. Thyroid Scans are Used for the Following Reasons

1. Identifying nodules and determining if they are "hot" or "cold".
2. Measuring the size of the goiter prior to treatment.
3. Follow-up of thyroid cancer patients after surgery.
4. Locating thyroid tissue outside the neck, i.e. base of the tongue or in the chest.

## 5.6. Relationship between Calcium, Phosphate and Vitamin D Metabolism

| Calcium | Phosphate | Due to |
|---------|-----------|--------|
| High | High | High levels of vitamin D |
| Low | Low | Low levels of vitamin D |
| High | Low | Hyperparathyroidism |
| Low | High | Hypoparathyroidism |

## 5.7. Differential Diagnosis of Rickets

| Type of Rickets | | Ca | Phos | Alk Phos | 25-OHD | 1, 25-OHD | PTH |
|---|---|---|---|---|---|---|---|
| Vit. D deficiency | Mild | NL, Low | NL, Low | High | Low | NL | NL |
| | Moderate | NL, Low | Low | Very high | Low | NL | High |
| | Severe | Low | Low | Very high | Very low | Low | Very high |
| F HR | | NL | Very low | High | NL | NL, Low | NL |
| Deficiency of | 25-OHase | NL | Low | High | Low | High | ? |
| | 1-alpha-OHase | Very low | Very low | Very high | NL | Low | Very high |
| Resist 1, 25-OH | | Very low | Very low | High | NL | Very high | High |

## 5.8. Insulin Therapy

| Type | Examples | Appearance | Onset | Peak | Duration |
|------|----------|------------|-------|------|----------|
| Rapid-acting | Apidra (insulin **Glulisine**) | Clear | 5–15 minutes | 30–60 minutes | 3–5 hours |
| | Humalog (insulin **Lispro**) | Clear | 5–15 minutes | 30–90 minutes | 3–5 hours |
| | Novolog (insulin **Aspart**) | Clear | 5–15 minutes | 40–50 minutes | 3–5 hours |

*Contd...*

*Contd...*

| Type | Examples | Appearance | Onset | Peak | Duration |
|---|---|---|---|---|---|
| **Short-acting** | Humulin-R (insulin **regular**) | Clear | 30 minutes | 1½–2 hours | 6–8 hours |
| **Intermediate-acting** | Humulin-N (insulin **NPH**) | Cloudy | 1–4 hours | 4–12 hours | 14–24 hours |
| **Long-acting** | Lantus (insulin **Glargine**) | Clear | 1–2 hours | Minimal peak | Upto 24 hours |
|  | Levemir (insulin **Detemir**) | Clear | 2 hours | Minimal peak | Upto 24 hours |

## 5.8. 1. Insulin therapy—Types, peak and duration

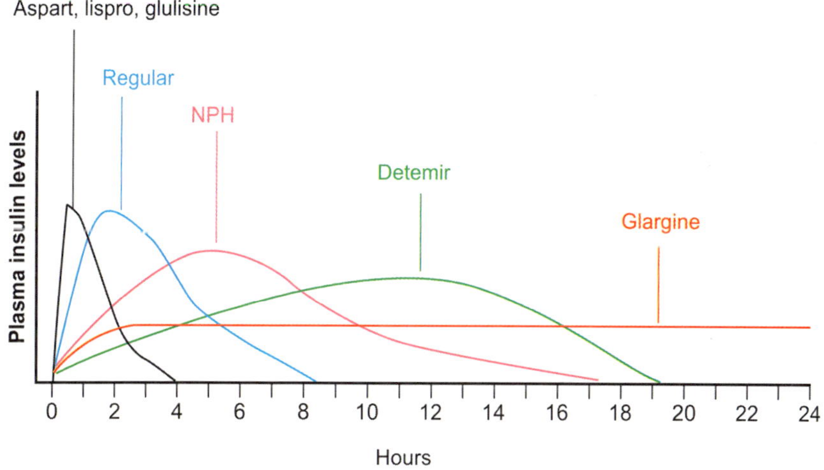


**Fig. 5.1**: Graph of types, peak and duration of various insulin therapy

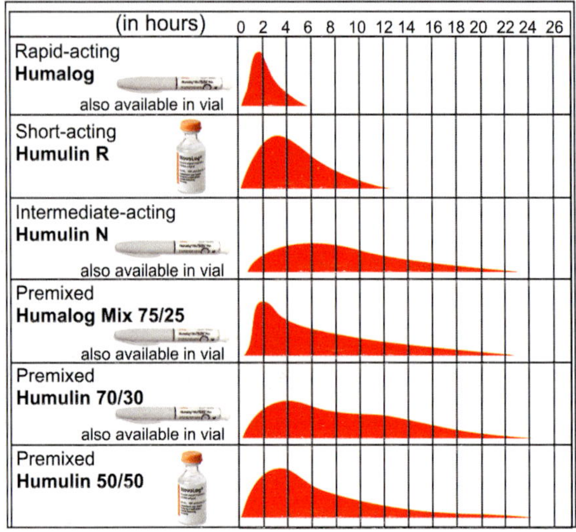


**Fig. 5.2**: Types, peak and duration of various insulin therapy

## Bibliography

1. http://emedicine.medscape.com
2. http://www.diabetes.co.uk
3. http://www.diabetes.org
4. http://www.endocrine.niddk.nih.gov

# Fluids, Electrolytes and Nutrition

## 6.1. Glucose in the Maintenance Fluids

- Provides approximately 20% of the normal caloric needs.
- Prevents the development of starvation ketoacidosis.
- Diminished the protein degradation that would occur if the patient received no calories.
- Provides added osmoles thus avoiding the administration of hypotonic fluids that may cause hemolysis.

## 6.2. Goals of Maintenance Fluids to Prevent

- Dehydration
- Electrolyte disorders
- Ketoacidosis
- Protein degradation.

## 6.3. Body Weight Method for Calculating Daily Maintenance Fluid Volume

| Body weight | Fluid per day |
|---|---|
| 0–10 kg | 100 mL/kg |
| 11–20 kg | 1,000 mL + 50 mL/kg for each kg > 10 kg |
| >20 kg | 1,500 mL + 20 mL/kg for each kg > 20 kg* |
| *The maximum total fluid per day is 2,400 mL | |

## 6.4. Hourly Maintenance Water Rate

| Body weight | Hourly maintenance water rate |
|---|---|
| 0–10 kg | 4 mL/kg/hour |
| 10–20 kg | 40 mL/hour + 2 mL/kg/hour × (wt. −10 kg) |
| >20 kg | 60 mL/hour + 1 mL/kg/hour × (wt. −20 kg)* |
| *The maximum fluid rate is normally 100 mL /hour | |

## 6.5. Composition of Intravenous Fluids

| Fluid | [Na$^+$] | [Cl$^-$] | [K$^+$] | [Ca$^{2+}$] | [Lactate$^-$] |
|---|---|---|---|---|---|
| Normal saline (0.9% NaCl) | 154 | 154 | | | |
| ½ Normal saline (0.45% NaCl) | 77 | 77 | | | |
| 0.2 Normal saline (0.2% NaCl) | 34 | 34 | | | |
| Ringer lactate | 130 | 109 | 4 | 3 | 28 |

## 6.6. Natural Sources of Water Loss

| Source | % |
|---|---|
| Urine | 60% |
| Insensible loss (skin and lung) | ~ 35% |
| Stool | 5% |

## 6.7. Adjustments in Maintenance Water

| Source | Causes of increased water needs | Causes of decreased water needs |
|---|---|---|
| Skin | | |
| | Radiant warmer | Incubator (premature infant) |
| | Phototherapy | |
| | Fever | |
| | Sweat | |
| | Burns | |
| Lungs | | |
| | Tachypnea | Humidified ventilator |
| | Tracheostomy | |
| Gastrointestinal tract | | |
| | Diarrhea | |
| | Emesis | |
| | Nasogastric suction | |
| Renal | | |
| | Polyuria | Oliguria/anuria |
| Miscellaneous | | |
| | Surgical drain | Hypothyroidism |
| | Third spacing | |

## 6.8. Replacement Fluid for Diarrhea

| Average composition of diarrhea | |
|---|---|
| Electrolyte | Amount |
| Sodium | 55 mEq/L |
| Potassium | 25 mEq/L |
| Bicarbonate | 15 mEq/L |
| Approach to replacement of ongoing losses | |
| • **Solution**: D5 0.2 normal saline +20 mEq/L sodium bicarbonate +20 mEq/L KCl | |
| • Replace stool mL/mL every 1–6 hours. | |

## 6.9. Replacement Fluid for Emesis or Nasogastric Losses

| Average composition of gastric fluid | |
|---|---|
| Electrolyte | Amount |
| Sodium | 60 mEq/L |
| Potassium | 10 mEq/L |
| Chloride | 90 mEq/L |
| Approach to replacement of ongoing losses | |
| • **Solution**:  Normal saline +10 mEq/L KCl | |
| • Replace output mL/mL every 1–6 hours. | |

## 6.10. Adjusting Fluid Therapy for Altered Renal Output

**Oliguria/Anuria**
- Place patient on insensible fluids (25–40% of maintenance)
- Replace urine output mL/mL with  ½ normal saline.

**Polyuria**
- Place patient on insensible fluids (25–40% of maintenance).
- Measure urine electrolytes.
- Replace output mL/mL with solution based on measured urine electrolytes.

## 6.11. Clinical Evaluation of Dehydration

### 6.11.1. Mild dehydration

**Mild dehydration (< 5% in an infant, <3% in an older child or adult)**
- Normal or increased pulse
- Decreased urine output
- Thirsty
- Normal physical findings.

### 6.11.2. Moderate dehydration

**Moderate dehydration (5–10% in an infant, 3–6% in an older child or adult)**
- Tachycardia
- Little or no urine output
- Irritable/lethargy
- Sunken eyes and fontanel
- Decreased tears
- Dry mucous membrane
- Mild delay in elasticity (skin turgor)
- Delay capillary refill (>1.5 sec)
- Cool and pale.

### 6.11.3. Severe dehydration

**Severe dehydration (>10% in an infant, >6% in an older child or adult)**
- Rapid and weak or absent peripheral pulses
- Decreased blood pressure
- No urine output
- Very sunken eyes and fontanel
- No tears
- Parched mucous membranes
- Delayed elasticity (poor skin turgor)
- Very delayed capillary refill (>3 sec)
- Cold and mottled
- Limp
- Depressed consciousness.

## 6.12. Fluid Management of Dehydration

### 6.12.1. Steps

**Step. 1**
- Restore intravascular volume
- Normal saline: 20 mL/kg over 20 minutes
- Repeat as needed.

**Step. 2**

- Rapid volume repletion: 20 mL/kg normal saline or Ringer lactate (maximum = 1L) over 2 hours.

**Step. 3**

- Calculate 24 hours fluid needs: Maintenance + deficit volume.

**Step. 4**

- Subtract isotonic fluid already administered from 24 hours fluid needs.

**Step. 5**

- Administer remaining volume over 24 hours. Using D5 ½ normal saline +20 mEq/L KCl.

**Step. 6**

- Replace ongoing losses as they occur.

## 6.13. Monitoring Therapy

- Vital signs
  - Pulse
  - Blood pressure.
- Intake and output
  - Fluid balance
  - Urine output and specific gravity.
- Physical examination
  - Weight
  - Clinical signs of depletion or overload.
- Electrolytes.

## 6.14. Treatment of Hypernatremic Dehydration

### 6.14.1. Steps

**Step. 1: Restore intravascular volume**
- Normal saline: 20 mL/kg over 20 minutes
- Repeat until intravascular volume restored.

**Step. 2: Determiner time for correction based on initial sodium**

**Step. 3: Administer fluid at constant rate over time for correction**

| Serum sodium | Time for correction |
| --- | --- |
| 145–157 mEq/L | 24 hours |
| 158–170 mEq/L | 48 hours |
| 171–183 mEq/L | 72 hours |
| 184–196 mEq/L | 84 hours |

- Typical fluid: D5 ½ normal saline (with 20 mEq/L KCl unless contraindicated).
- Typical rate: 1.25–1.5 times maintenance.

**Step. 4: Follow serum sodium concentration**

**Step. 5: Adjust fluid based on clinical status and serum sodium concentration**

- Signs of volume depletion: Administer normal saline 20 mEq/kg
- Sodium decreases too rapidly:
  - Increase sodium concentration of intravenous fluid
  - Decrease rate of intravenous fluid.
- Sodium decreases too slowly:
  - Decrease sodium concentration of intravenous fluid
  - Increase rate of intravenous fluid.

**Step. 6: Replace ongoing losses as they occur**

## 6.15. Treatment of Hyponatremic Dehydration

### 6.15.1. Steps

**Step. 1: Restore intravascular volume**

- The initial goal in treating hyponatremia is correction of intravascular volume depletion with isotonic fluid (NS or LR).
- An overcorrection in the serum sodium concentration (>135 mEq/L) is associated with an increased risk of central pontine myelinolysis (CPM).
- The risk of CPM also increased with overly rapid correction of the serum sodium concentration.
- It is best to avoid increasing the sodium >12 mEq/L each 24 hours.
- Patients with neurologic symptoms (seizures) as a result of hyponatremia need to receive an acute infusion of hypertonic (3%) saline to increase the serum sodium concentration rapidly.

**Step. 2: Notes**

- Each mL/kg of 3% sodium chloride increases the serum sodium by approximately 1 mEq/L.
- A child with active symptoms often improves after receiving 4–6 mL/kg of 3% sodium chloride.

## 6.16. A Guideline for Oral Rehydration

| Mild dehydration | 50 mL /kg of the oral rehydration solution (ORS) | Given within 4 hours |
|---|---|---|
| Moderate dehydration | 100 mL/kg (ORS) | Over 4 hours |
| Additional | 10 mL/kg (ORS) | For each stool |

## 6.17. Composition of Oral Rehydration Solutions (ORS)

| Solution | Glucose (mmol/L) | Na$^+$ (mEq/L) | K$^+$ (mEq/L) | Cl$^-$ (mEq/L) | Base (mEq/L) | Osmolality (mOsm/kg) |
|---|---|---|---|---|---|---|
| WHO solution | 111 | 90 | 20 | 80 | 30 | 311 |
| Rehydralyte | 140 | 75 | 20 | 65 | 30 | 310 |
| Pedialyte | 140 | 45 | 20 | 35 | 30 | 250 |
| Pediatric electrolyte | 140 | 45 | 20 | 35 | 55 | 250 |
| Infalyte | 70* | 50 | 25 | 45 | 34 | 200 |
| Naturalyte | 140 | 45 | 20 | 35 | 55 | 238 |

*Rice syrup solids are the carbohydrate source

## 6.18. Composition of Oral Rehydration Salts Solution for Severely Malnourished Children (ReSoMal)

| Component | Concentration (mmol/L) |
|---|---|
| Glucose | 125 |
| Sodium | 45 |
| Potassium | 40 |
| Chloride | 70 |
| Citrate | 7 |
| Magnesium | 3 |
| Zinc | 0.3 |
| Copper | 0.045 |
| Osmolarity | 300 |

## 6.19. Causes of Hypernatremia

1. **Excess sodium**
   - Improperly mixed formula.
   - Excess sodium bicarbonate.
   - Ingestion of seawater or sodium chloride.
   - Intentional salt poisoning (child abuse or Munchausen syndrome by proxy).
   - Intravenous hypertonic saline.
   - Hyperaldosteronism.
2. **Water deficit**
   - Nephrogenic diabetes insipidus
     - Acquired
     - X-linked
     - Autosomal recessive
     - Autosomal dominant.
   - Central diabetes insipidus:
     - Acquired
     - Autosomal recessive
     - Autosomal dominant
     - Wolfram syndrome.
   - Increased insensible losses:
     - Premature infants
     - Radiant warmers
     - Phototherapy.
   - Inadequate intake:
     - Ineffective breastfeeding
     - Child neglect or abuse
     - Adipsia (lack of thirst).
3. **Water and sodium deficit**
   - Gastrointestinal losses:
     - Diarrhea
     - Emesis/nasogastric suction
     - Osmotic cathartics (lactulose).
   - Cutaneous losses:
     - Burns
     - Excessive sweating.
   - Renal losses:
     - Osmotic diuretics (mannitol)
     - Diabetes mellitus
     - Chronic kidney disease (dysplasia and obstructive uropathy)
     - Polyuric phase of acute tubular necrosis.
   - Postobstructive diuresis.

## 6.20. Causes of Hyponatremia

1. **Extrarenal losses**
   - Gastrointestinal (emesis and diarrhea)
   - Skin (sweating or burns)
   - (Third space losses).
2. **Renal losses**
   - Thiazide or loop diuretics
   - Osmotic diuresis
   - Postobstructive diuresis
   - Polyuric phase of acute tubular necrosis
   - Juvenile nephronophthisis
   - Autosomal recessive polycystic kidney disease
   - Tubulointerstitial nephritis
   - Obstructive uropathy
   - Cerebral salt wasting
   - Proximal (type II) renal tubular acidosis
   - Lack of aldosterone effect (high serum potassium):
     - Absence of aldosterone (e.g. 21-hydroxylase deficiency)
     - Pseudohypoaldosteronism type I
     - Urinary tract obstruction and/or infection.
3. **Euvolemic hyponatremia**
   - Syndrome of inappropriate antidiuretic hormone secretion
   - Nephrogenic syndrome of inappropriate antidiuresis
   - Desmopressin acetate
   - Glucocorticoid deficiency
   - Hypothyroidism
   - Water intoxication:
     - Iatrogenic (excess hypotonic intravenous fluids)
     - Feeding infants excessive water products
     - Swimming lessons
     - Tap water enema
     - Child abuse
     - Psychogenic polydipsia
     - Diluted formula.
4. **Hypovolemic hyponatremia**
   - Congestive heart failure.
   - Cirrhosis.
   - Nephrotic syndrome.
   - Renal failure.
   - Capillary leak due to sepsis.
   - Hypoalbuminemia due to gastrointestinal disease (protein-losing enteropathy).

## 6.21. Causes of Hyperkalemia

1. **Transcellular shifts**
   - Acidosis
   - Rhabdomyolysis
   - Tumorlysis syndrome
   - Tissue necrosis
   - Hemolysis/hematomas/gastrointestinal bleeding
   - Malignant hyperthermia
   - Hyperkalemic periodic paralysis
   - Succinylcholine
   - Digitalis intoxication
   - Fluoride intoxication
   - $\alpha$-adrenergic blockers
   - Insulin deficiency
   - Hyperosmolality
   - Exercise.
2. **Decreased excretion**
   - Renal failure
   - Hyporeninemic hypoaldosteronism:
     - Urinary tract obstruction
     - Sickle cell disease
     - Kidney transplant
     - Lupus nephritis
   - Primary adrenal disease:
     - Acquired Addison disease
     - 21-hydroxylase deficiency
     - 3$\alpha$-hydroxysteroid dehydrogenase deficiency
     - Lipoid congenital adrenal hyperplasia
     - Adrenal hypoplasia congenita
     - Aldosterone synthase deficiency
     - Adrenoleukodystrophy.
   - Renal tubular disease:
     - Pseudohypoaldosteronism type I
     - Pseudohypoaldosteronism type II
     - Bartter syndrome, type II
     - Urinary tract obstruction
     - Sickle cell disease.
   - Medications:
     - Angiotensin II blockers
     - Potassium-sparing diuretics

- Calcineurin inhibitors
- Nonsteroidal anti-inflammatory drugs
- Trimethoprim
- Heparin.

## 6.22. Causes of Hypokalemia

1. **Transcellular shifts**
   - Alkalemia.
   - Insulin.
   - $\alpha$-adrenergic agonists.
   - Hypokalemic periodic paralysis.
   - Thyrotoxic period paralysis.
   - Refeeding syndrome.
   - Drugs/toxins (theophylline, barium, toluene, cesium chloride, hydroxychloroquine).
2. **Decreased intake**
   - Anorexia nervosa.
3. **External losses**
   - Diarrhea
   - Laxative abuse
   - Sweating
   - Sodium polystyrene sulfonate (kayexalate) or clay ingestion.
4. **Renal losses**
   - With metabolic acidosis
   - Without specific acid-base disturbance
   - With metabolic alkalosis:
     - Low urine chloride
     - High urine chloride and normal blood pressure
     - High urine chloride and high blood pressure.
   - Licorice ingestion
   - Liddle syndrome.
   4.1. **With metabolic acidosis**
      - Distal renal tubular acidosis
      - Proximal renal tubular acidosis
      - Ureterosigmoidostomy
      - Diabetic ketoacidosis.
   4.2. **Without specific acid-base disturbance**
      - Tubular toxins: Amphotericin, cisplatin, aminoglycosides
      - Interstitial nephritis
      - Diuretic phase of acute tubular necrosis
      - Postobstructive diuresis

- Hypomagnesemia
- High urine anions (e.g. penicillin or penicillin derivatives).

4.3. **With metabolic alkalosis**
- Low urine chloride
    - Emesis or nasogastric suction
    - Chloride-losing diarrhea
    - Cystic fibrosis
    - Low-chloride formula
    - Posthypercapnia
    - Previous loop or thiazide diuretic use.
- High urine chloride and normal blood pressure
    - Gitelman syndrome.
    - Bartter syndrome.
    - Autosomal dominant hypoparathyroidism.
    - EAST syndrome (epilepsy, ataxia, sensorineural hearing loss, and tubulopathy).
    - Loop and thiazide diuretics.
- High urine chloride and high blood pressure
    - Adrenal adenoma or hyperplasia
    - Glucocorticoid-remediable aldosteronism
    - Renovascular disease
    - Renin-secreting tumor
    - $17\alpha$-hydroxylase deficiency
    - $11\alpha$-hydroxylase deficiency
    - Cushing syndrome
    - $11\alpha$-hydroxysteroid dehydrogenase deficiency.

## 6.23. Causes of Hypercalcemia

1. Infant with subcutaneous fat necrosis
2. Hypophosphatasia
3. Idiopathic hypercalcemia of infancy
4. Williams syndrome (10%)
5. Hypervitaminosis D
6. Prolonged immobilization
7. Jansen-type metaphyseal chodrodysplasia.

## 6.24. Causes of Hyperphosphatemia

1. **Transcellular shifts**
- Tumor-lysis syndrome
- Rhabdomyolysis
- Acute hemolysis
- Diabetic ketoacidosis and lactic acidosis.

2. **Increased intake**
   - Enemas and laxatives
   - Cow's milk in infants
   - Treatment of hypophosphatemia
   - Vitamin D intoxication.
3. **Decreased excretion**
   - Renal failure
   - Hypoparathyroidism or pseudohypoparathyroidism
   - Acromegaly
   - Hyperthyroidism
   - Tumoral calcinosis with hyperphosphatemia.

## 6.25. Causes of Hypophosphatemia

1. **Transcellular shifts**
   - Glucose infusion
   - Insulin
   - Refeeding
   - Total parenteral nutrition
   - Respiratory alkalosis
   - Tumor growth
   - Bone marrow transplantation
   - Hungry bone syndrome.
2. **Decreased intake**
   - Nutritional
   - Premature infants
   - Low phosphorus formula
   - Antacids and other phosphate binders.
3. **Renal losses**
   - Hyperparathyroidism
   - Parathyroid hormone-related peptide
   - X-linked hypophosphatemic rickets
   - Tumor-induced osteomalacia
   - Autosomal dominant hypophosphatemic rickets
   - Autosomal recessive hypophosphatemic rickets
   - Fanconi syndrome
   - Dent disease
   - Hypophosphatemic rickets with hypercalciuria
   - Hypophosphatemic nephrolithiasis/osteoporosis type I
   - Hypophosphatemic nephrolithiasis/osteoporosis type II
   - Volume expansion and intravenous fluids
   - Metabolic acidosis

- Diuretics
- Glycosuria
- Glucocorticoids
- Kidney transplantation.
4. **Multifactorial**
   - Vitamin D deficiency
   - Vitamin D-dependent rickets type I
   - Vitamin D-dependent rickets type II
   - Sepsis.

## 6.26. Causes of Hypomagnesemia

1. **Gastrointestinal disorders**
   - Diarrhea
   - Nasogastric suction or emesis
   - Inflammatory bowel disease
   - Celiac disease
   - Cystic fibrosis
   - Intestinal lymphangiectasia
   - Small bowel resection or bypass
   - Pancreatitis
   - Protein-calorie malnutrition
   - Hypomagnesemia with secondary hypocalcemia.
2. **Renal disorders**
   - **Medications**
     - Amphotericin
     - Cisplatin
     - Cyclosporin
     - Loop diuretics
     - Mannitol
     - Pentamidine
     - Aminoglycosided
     - Thiazide diuretics.
   - **Chronic kidney diseases**
     - Interstitial nephritis
     - Glomerulonephritis
     - Postrenal transplantation.
   - **Associated diseases**
     - Diabetes
     - Acute tubular necrosis (recovery phase)
     - Postobstructive nephropathy
     - Primary aldosteronism

- Hypercalcemia
- Intravenous fluids.
- **Genetic diseases**
  - Gitelman syndrome.
  - Bartter syndrome.
  - Familial hypomagnesemia with hypercalciuria and nephrocalcinosis.
  - Familial hypomagnesemia with hypercalciuria, nephrocalcinosis, and severe ocular involvement.
  - Autosomal recessive renal magnesium wasting with normocal-ciuria.
  - Autosomal dominant renal magnesium wasting.
  - Renal cysts and diabetes syndrome.
  - EAST syndrome.
  - Autosomal dominant hypoparathyroidism.
  - Mitochondrial disorders.
- **Miscellaneous causes**
  - Poor intake
  - Hungry bone syndrome
  - Insulin administration
  - Pancreatitis
  - Intrauterine growth retardation
  - Infants of diabetic mothers
  - Exchange transfusion.

## 6.27. Systematic Evaluation of an Arterial Blood Gas Sample

1. Assessment of an arterial blood gas sample requires knowledge of normal values:

| | |
|---|---|
| pH | 7.35–7.45 |
| $[HCO_3^-]$ | 20–28 mEq/L |
| $PCO_2$ | 35–45 mmHg |

2. In most cases, this is accomplished via a 3-step process
   - Determine whether acidemia or alkalemia is present
   - Determine a cause of the acidemia or alkalemia
   - Determine whether a mixed disorder is present.
3. Definitions
   - Acidemia: It is a pH below normal (<7.35).
   - Alkalemia: It is a pH above normal (>7.45).

- Metabolic acidosis have a low serum bicarbonate concentration.
- Metabolic alkalosis: The serum bicarbonate concentration is increased.
- Respiratory acidosis: It is an inappropriate increase in blood carbon dioxide ($PCO_2$).
- Respiratory alkalosis: It is an inappropriate reduction in the blood carbon dioxide concentration.

4. The plasma anion gap
   - It is useful for evaluating patients with a metabolic acidosis.
   - It divides patients into 2 diagnostic groups, those with normal anion gap and those with increased anion gap.
   - The following formula determines the anion gap.

$$\text{Anion gap} = [Na^+] - [Cl^-] - [HCO_3^-]$$

## 6.28. Plasma Osmolality

The plasma osmolality can be estimated by a calculation based on the following formula:

$$\text{Osmolality} = 2\times [Na] + [glucose]/18 + [BUN]/2.8$$

## 6.29. Basic Mechanisms of a Metabolic Acidosis

Metabolic acidosis occur via 3 basic mechanisms:
1. Loss of bicarbonate from the body
2. Impaired ability to excrete acid by the kidney
3. Addition of acid to the body (exogenous or endogenous).

## 6.30. Causes of Metabolic Acidosis

I. **Normal anion gap**
   Diarrhea
   Renal tubular acidosis (RTA):
   1. Distal (type I) RTA
   2. Proximal (type II) RTA
   3. Hyperkalemic (type IV) RTA
   Urinary tract diversions
   Posthypocapnia
   Ammonium chloride intake.

II. **Increased anion gap**
   1. Lactic acidosis:
      Tissue hypoxia:
      – Shock
      – Hypoxemia
      – Severe anemia
      Liver failure

Malignancy
Intestinal bacterial overgrowth
Inborn errors of metabolism
Medications:
– Nucleoside reverse transcriptase inhibitors
– Metformin
– Propofol.
2. Ketoacidosis:
   – Diabetic ketoacidosis
   – Starvation ketoacidosis
   – Alcoholic ketoacidosis
   – Kidney failure.
3. Poisoning:
   – Ethylene glycol
   – Methanol
   – Salicylate
   – Toluene
   – Paraldehyde.
4. Inborn errors of metabolism

## 6.31. Causes of Metabolic Alkalosis

I. Chloride-responsive (urinary chloride < 15 mEq/L)
   Gastric loss:
   • Emesis
   • Nasogastric suction
   Diuretics (loop or thiazide)
   Chloride-losing diarrhea
   Chloride-deficient formula
   Cystic fibrosis
   Posthypercapnia.
II. Chloride-resistant (urinary chloride > 20 mEq/L)
   1. High blood pressure:
      • Adrenal adenoma or hyperplasia
      • Glucocorticoid-remediable aldosteronism
      • Renovascular disease
      • Renin-secreting tumor
      • $17\alpha$-hydroxylase deficiency
      • $11\alpha$-hydroxylase deficiency
      • Cushing syndrome
      • $11\alpha$-hydroxysteroid dehydrogenase deficiency
      • Licorice ingestion
      • Liddle syndrome.

2.  Normal blood pressure:
    Gitelman syndrome
    Bartter syndrome
    Autosomal dominant hypoparathyroidism
    EAST syndrome
    Base administration.

## 6.32. Causes of Respiratory Acidosis

| I.   Central nervous system depression | |
| --- | --- |
| Encephalitis | Stroke |
| Head trauma | Hypoxic brain damage |
| Brain tumor | Obesity-hypoventilation (Pickwickian syndrome) |
| Central sleep apnea | Increased intracranial pressure |
| Primary pulmonary hypoventilation | Medications: |
| | • Narcotics |
| | • Benzodiazepines |
| | • Barbiturates |

| II.   Disorder of the spinal cord peripheral nerves, or  neuromuscular junction | |
| --- | --- |
| Diaphragmatic paralysis | Botulism |
| Guillain-Barré syndrome | Myasthenia |
| Poliomyelitis | Multiple sclerosis |
| Spinal muscular atrophies | Spinal cord injury |
| Tick paralysis | Medications: |
| | • Vecuronium |
| | • Aminoglycosides |
| | • Organophosphates |

| III.   Respiratory muscle weakness | |
| --- | --- |
| Muscular dystrophy | Hypokalemia |
| Hypothyroidism | Hypophosphatemia |
| Malnutrition | Medications: |
| | • Succinylcholine |
| | • Corticosteroids |

| IV. Pulmonary diseases | |
| --- | --- |
| Pneumonia | Adult respiratory distress syndrome |
| Pneumothorax | Neonatal respiratory distress syndrome |
| Asthma | Cystic fibrosis |
| Bronchiolitis | Bronchopulmonary dysplasia |
| Pulmonary edema | Meconium aspiration |
| Pulmonary hemorrhage | Pulmonary thromboembolus |
| Interstitial fibrosis | |

| V. Upper airway diseases | |
| --- | --- |
| Aspiration | Tonsillar hypertrophy |
| Laryngospasm | Vocal cord paralysis |
| Angioedema | Extrinsic tumor |
| Obstructive sleep apnea | Extrinsic or intrinsic hemangioma |

| VI. Miscellaneous | |
| --- | --- |
| Flail chest | Kyphoscoliosis |
| Cardiac arrest | Decreased diaphragmatic movement due to ascites or peritoneal dialysis |

## 6.33. Causes of Respiratory Alkalosis

| I. Hypoxemia or tissue hypoxia | |
| --- | --- |
| Pneumonia | Laryngospasm |
| Pulmonary edema | Aspiration |
| Cyanotic heart disease | Carbon monoxide poisoning |
| Congestive heart failure | Pulmonary embolism |
| Asthma | Interstitial lung disease |
| Severe anemia | Hypotension |
| High altitude | |

| II. Lung receptor stimulation | |
| --- | --- |
| Pneumonia | Hemothorax |
| Pulmonary edema | Pneumothorax |
| Asthma | Pulmonary embolism |
| Respiratory distress syndrome (adult or infant) | |

| III. | Central stimulation | |
|---|---|---|
| | 1. Central nervous system disease: | |
| | Subarachnoid hemorrhage | |
| | Encephalitis or meningitis | |
| | Trauma | |
| | Brain tumor | |
| | Stroke | |
| | 2. Other causes | |
| | Fever | Sepsis |
| | Pain | Mechanical ventilation |
| | Anxiety (panic attack) | Hyperammonemia |
| | Psychogenic hyperventilation or anxiety | Extracorporeal membrane oxygenation or hemodialysis |
| | Liver failure | |
| | Medications: | |
| | • Salicylate intoxication | |
| | • Theophylline | |
| | • Progesterone | |
| | • Exogenous catecholamines | |
| | • Caffeine | |

## 6.34. Causes of Rickets

| I. | Vitamin D disorders |
|---|---|
| | 1. Nutritional vitamin D deficiency |
| | 2. Congenital vitamin D deficiency |
| | 3. Secondary vitamin D deficiency: |
| | • Malabsorption |
| | • Increased degradation |
| | • Decreased liver 25-hydroxylase |
| | 4. Vitamin D-dependent rickets type I |
| | 5. Vitamin D-dependent rickets type II |
| | 6. Chronic renal failure |

II.  Calcium deficiency

1.  Low intake:
- Diet
- Premature infants (rickets of prematurity)
2.  Malabsorption:
- Primary disease
- Dietary inhibitors of calcium absorption

III.  Phosphorus  deficiency

1.  Inadequate intake
- Premature infants (rickets of prematurity)
- Aluminum-containing antacids

IV.  Renal losses

1.  X-linked hypophosphatemic rickets
2.  Autosomal dominant hypophosphatemic rickets
3.  Autosomal recessive hypophosphatemic rickets
4.  Hereditary hypophosphatemic rickets with hypercalciuria
5.  Overproduction of phosphatonin:
- Tumor-induced rickets
- McCune-Albright syndrome
- Epidermal nevus syndrome
- Neurofibromatosis
6.  Fanconi syndrome
7.  Dent disease
8.  Distal renal tubular acidosis

## 6.35.  Absolute and Relative Contraindications to Breastfeeding due to Maternal Conditions

1.  HIV and HTLV infection
- In the USA, breastfeeding is contraindicated.
- In other settings, health risks of not breastfeeding must be weighed against the risk of transmitting virus to the infant.
2.  Tuberculosis infection
- Breastfeeding is contraindicated until completion of approximately 2 week of appropriate maternal therapy.
3.  Varicella-zoster infection
- Infant should not have direct contact to active lesions
- Infant should receive immune globulin.

4. Herpes simplex infection
   - Breastfeeding is contraindicated with active herpetic lesions of the breast.
5. CMV infection
   - May be found in milk of mothers who are CMV seropositive
   - Transmission through human milk
   - Causing symptomatic illness in term infants is uncommon.
6. Hepatitis B infection
   - Infants routinely receive hepatitis B immune globulin and hepatitis B vaccine if mother is HbsAg positive.
   - No delay in initiation of breastfeeding is required.
7. Hepatitis C infection
   - Breastfeeding is not contraindicated.
8. Cigaret smoking
   - Discourage cigaret smoking, but smoking is not a contraindication to breastfeeding.
9. Chemotherapy and radiopharmaceuticals
   - Breastfeeding is generally contraindicated.

## 6.36. Formula Feeding

### 6.36.1. Facts

- Infant formulas are available in:
  - Ready-to-feed
  - Concentrated liquid
  - Powder forms.
- Ready-to-feed products generally provide 20 kcal/30 mL (1 oz).

### 6.36.2. Cow's milk protein-based formulas

- Intact cow's milk-based formulas contain a protein concentration varying from 1.45–1.6 gm/dL
  {Considerably higher than in mature breast milk (~1 gm/dL)}.
- The whey : casein ratio varies from 18 : 82–60 : 40 .
- The predominant whey protein is $\alpha$-globulin in bovine milk
  {$\alpha$-lactalbumin in human milk}.
- Plant or a mixture of plant and animal oils are the source of fat in infant formulas, and fat provides 40–50% of the energy in cow's milk-based formulas.
- Lactose is the major carbohydrate in mother's milk and in standard cow's milk-based infant formulas for term infants.

### 6.36.3. Soy formulas

- Soy protein-based formulas on the market are all free of cow's milk protein and lactose and provide 67 kcal/dL.
- The protein is a soy isolate supplemented with l-methionine, l-carnitine, and taurine to provide a protein content of 2.45–2.8 gm per 100 kcal.
- The fat content is 5.0–5.5 gm per 100 kcal or 3.4–3.6 gm/dL. The oils used include soy, palm, sunflower, olein, safflower and coconut. DHA and ARA are now added routinely.
- Indications include galactosemia and hereditary lactase deficiency.
- The routine use of soy protein-based formula has no proven value in the prevention or management of infantile colic, fussiness, or atopic disease.
- Infants with documented cow's milk protein-induced enteropathy or enterocolitis often are also sensitive to soy protein and should not be given isolated soy protein-based formula.

### 6.36.4. Protein hydrolysate formula

Protein hydrolysate formulas may be:
1. Partially hydrolyzed, containing oligopeptides with a molecular weight of <5000 d.
2. Extensively hydrolyzed, containing peptides with a molecular weight <3000 d.

1. **Partially hydrolyzed proteins**
   - Have fat blends similar to cow's milk-based formulas.
   - Carbohydrates are supplied by corn maltodextrin or corn syrup solids

     – Because the protein is not extensively hydrolyzed, these formulas should not be fed to infants who are allergic to cow's milk protein.
2. **Extensively hydrolyzed formulas**
   - May be more effective than partially hydrolyzed in preventing atopic disease.
   - Extensively hydrolyzed formulas are the preferred formulas for infants intolerant to cow's milk or soy proteins
     – These formulas are lactose-free and can include medium-chain triglycerides.
     – They are useful in infants with gastrointestinal malabsorption due to:
       1. Cystic fibrosis
       2. Short gut syndrome
       3. Prolonged diarrhea.

## 6.36.5. Amino acid formulas

- Amino acid formulas are peptide-free formulas that contain mixtures of essential and nonessential amino acids.
- They are specifically designed for infants with dairy protein allergy who failed to thrive on extensively hydrolyzed protein formulas.

## 6.37. Endocrine Causes of Obesity

| Disease | Symptoms | | Laboratory tests |
|---|---|---|---|
| 1. **Cushing syndrome** | • Central obesity<br>• Hirsutism | • Moon face<br>• Hypertension | Dexametha-sone suppression test |
| 2. **Growth hormone deficiency** | • Short stature | • Slow linear growth | • Evoked GH response<br>• IGF-1 |
| 3. **Hyperinsulinism** | • Nesidioblastosis<br>• Pancreatic adenoma | • Hypoglycemia<br>• Mauriac syndrome | Insulin level |
| 4. **Hypothyroidism** | • Short stature<br>• Weight gain<br>• Fatigue | • Constipation<br>• Cold intolerance<br>• Myxedema | • TSH<br>• FT4 |
| 5. **Pseudo-hypoparathyroidism** | • Short metacarpals<br>• Subcutaneous calcifications<br>• Dysmorphic facies | • Mental retardation<br>• Short stature<br>• Hypocalcemia<br>• Hyperphosphatemia | Urine cAMP after synthetic PTH infusion |

## 6.38. Genetic Causes of Obesity

| Disease | Symptoms | | Laboratory tests |
|---|---|---|---|
| 1. Alstrom syndrome | • Cognitive impairment<br>• Retinitis pigmentosa<br>• Diabetes mellitus | • Hearing loss<br>• Hypogonadism<br>• Retinal degeneration | ALMS1 gene |
| 2. Bardet-Biedl syndrome | • Retinitis pigmentosa<br>• Renal abnormalities | • Polydactyly<br>• Hypogonadism | BBS1 gene |

*Contd...*

*Contd...*

| Disease | Symptoms | | Laboratory tests |
|---|---|---|---|
| 3. Biemond syndrome | • Cognitive impairment<br>• Iris coloboma | • Hypogonadism<br>• Polydactyly | |
| 4. Carpenter syndrome | • Polydactyly<br>• Syndactyly<br>• Cranial synostosis<br>• Mental retardation | | Mutations in the RAB23 gene, located on chromosome 6 in humans |
| 5. Down syndrome | • Short stature<br>• Dysmorphic facies<br>• Mental retardation | | Mutations in the VPS13B gene (often called the COH1 gene) at locus 8q22 |
| 6. Cohen syndrome | • Midchildhood-onset obesity<br>• Short stature<br>• Prominent maxillary incisors | • Hypotonia<br>• Mental retardation<br>• Microcephaly<br>• Decreased visual activity | Mutations in the VPS13B gene (often called the COH1 gene) at locus 8q22 |
| 7. Frohlich syndrome | Hypothalamic tumor | | |
| 8. Prader-Willi Syndrome | • Neonatal hypotonia<br>• Slow infant growth<br>• Small hands and feet<br>• Mental retardation<br>• Hypogonadism | • Hyperphagia leading to severe obesity<br>• Paradoxically elevated ghrelin | Partial deletion of chromosome 15 or loss of paternally expressed genes |
| 9. Turner syndrome | • Ovarian dysgenesis<br>• Lymphedema<br>• Web neck | • Short stature<br>• Cognitive impairment | XO chromosome |

## Bibliography


1. http://ajcn.nutrition.org
2. http://emedicine.medscape.com
3. http://web.squ.edu.om
4. http://www.cdc.gov

# Gastroenterology

## 7.1. Causes of Oropharyngeal Dysphagia

### 7.1.1. Neuromuscular disorders

1. Cerebral palsy
2. Brain tumors
3. Cerebrovascular accidents
4. Polio and postpolio syndromes
5. Multiple sclerosis
6. Myositis
7. Dermatomyositis
8. Myasthenia gravis
9. Muscular dystrophies.

### 7.1.2. Metabolic and autoimmune disorders

1. Hyperthyroidism
2. Systemic lupus erythematosus
3. Sarcoidosis
4. Amyloidosis.

### 7.1.3. Infectious diseases

1. Meningitis
2. Botulism
3. Diphtheria
4. Lyme disease
5. Neurosyphilis
6. Viral infections, e.g. polio, coxsackievirus, herpes and cytomegalovirus.

### 7.1.4. Structural lesions

1. Inflammatory: Abscess, pharyngitis
2. Congenital web
3. Cricopharyngeal bar
4. Dental problems
5. Bullous skin lesions
6. Plummer-Vinson syndrome
7. Zenker diverticulum
8. Extrinsic compression: Osteophytes, lymph nodes and thyroid swelling.

### 7.1.5. Others

1. Corrosive injury
2. After surgery
3. Side effects of medications
4. After radiation therapy.

## 7.2. Causes of Esophageal Dysphagia

### 7.2.1. Neuromuscular disorders

1. GERD
2. Diffuse esophageal spasm
3. Achalasia cardia
4. Scleroderma.

### 7.2.2. Mechanical

1. Intrinsic lesions
2. Foreign bodies
3. Esophagitis: GERD and eosinophilic esophagitis
4. Stricture: Corrosive injury, pill-induced and peptic
5. Esophageal webs
6. Esophageal rings
7. Esophageal diverticula
8. Neoplasm
9. Extrinsic lesions
10. Vascular compression
11. Mediastinal lesion
12. Cervical osteochondritis
13. Vertebral abnormalities.

## 7.3. Acid-base Imbalance

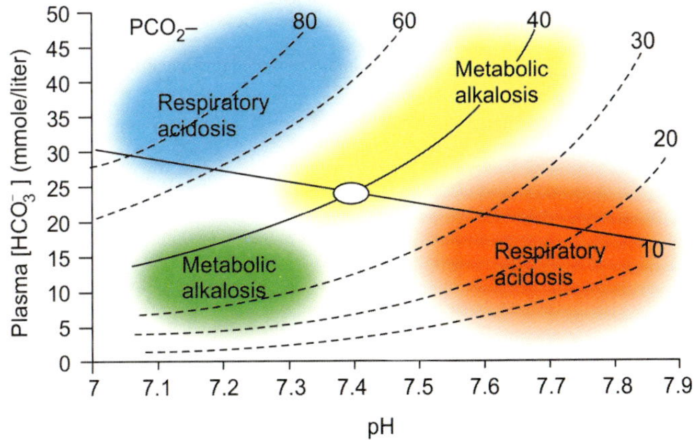



**Fig. 7.1**: Acid-base imbalance

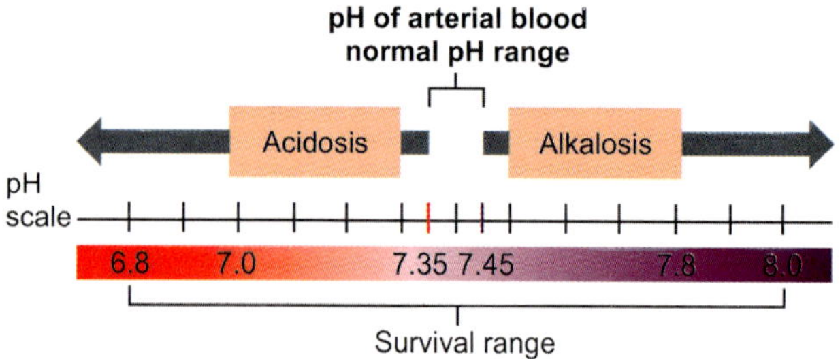


**Fig. 7.2**: pH scale

## 7.4. First and Second Lines of Defense Against pH Shift

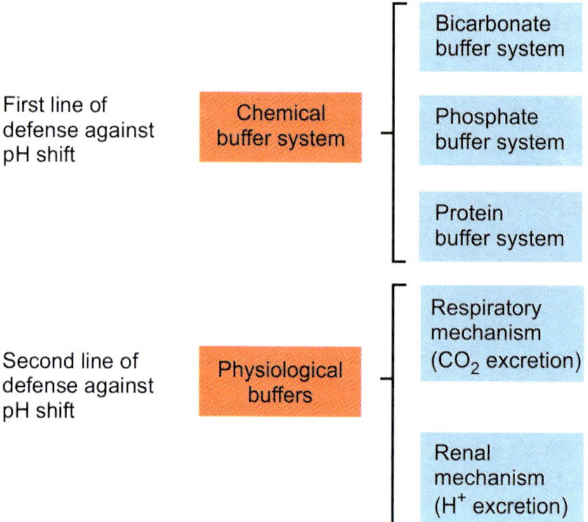


## 7.5. Derangement in Acid-base Balance

### 7.5.1. Metabolic acidosis

$\downarrow HCO_3^-$ and $\downarrow pH$

- Increased anion gap
    1. Lactic acidosis
    2. Ketoacidosis
    3. Drug poisoning (e.g. aspirin, ethylene, glycol and methanol).
- Normal anion gap
    1. Diarrhea
    2. Some kidney problems (e.g. renal tubular acidosis and interstitial nephritis).

### 7.5.2. Metabolic alkalosis

$\uparrow HCO_3^-$ and $\uparrow$ pH
- Chloride responsive (responds to NaCl or KCl therapy)
    1. Contraction alkalosis
    2. Diuretics
    3. Corticosteroids
    4. Gastric suctioning
    5. Vomiting.
- Chloride resistant
    1. Any hyperaldosterone state (e.g. Cushing's syndrome and Bartter's syndrome and severe $K^+$ depletion).

### 7.5.3. Respiratory acidosis

$\uparrow PaCO_2$ and $\downarrow$ pH
- Central nervous system depression (e.g. drug overdose).
- Chest bellows dysfunction (e.g. Guillain-Barré syndrome and myasthenia gravis).
- Disease of lungs and/or upper airway (e.g. chronic obstructive lung disease).

### 7.5.4. Respiratory alkalosis

$\downarrow PaCO_2$ and $\uparrow$ pH
- Hypoxemia (includes altitude)
- Anxiety
- Sepsis
- Any acute pulmonary insult (e.g. pneumonia, mild asthma attack, early pulmonary edema and pulmonary embolism).

## 7.6. Diagnosis of Acid-base Imbalances

1. Look at the pH
   Is it the primary problem acidosis (low) or alkalosis (high).
2. Check the $CO_2$ (respiratory indicator)
   Is it less than 35 (alkalosis) or more than 45 (acidosis).
3. Check the $HCO_3^-$ (metabolic indicator)
   Is it less than 22 (acidosis) or more than 26 (alkalosis).
4. Which is primary disorder (respiratory or metabolic)?
   If the pH is low (acidosis) $\rightarrow$ look to see: If $CO_2$ (more than 45) or $HCO_3^-$ (less than 22) is the indicator of acidosis (whichever is acidosis will be primary).
   If the pH is high (alkalosis) $\rightarrow$ look to see: If $CO_2$ (less than 35) or $HCO_3^-$ (more than 26) is the indicator alkalosis (whichever is alkalosis is the

primary). The one that matches the pH (acidosis or alkalosis), is the primary disorder.

## 7.7. Easy Blood Gas Interpretation

- pH high (alkalosis) or pH low (acidosis)
- High $pCO_2$ is respiratory acidosis
- Low $HCO_3^-$ is metabolic acidosis
- Look at the value that doesn't correspond to the observed pH change:
  - If it is inside the normal range, there is no compensation occurring.
  - If it is outside the normal range, the body is partially compensating for the problem, i.e. compensation-attempt to normalize pH.

## 7.8. Compensation-attempt to Normalize pH

| Primary problem | Compensation |
|---|---|
| • Respiratory acidosis | • Metabolic alkalosis |
| • Respiratory alkalosis | • Metabolic acidosis |
| • Metabolic acidosis | • Respiratory alkalosis |
| • Metabolic  alkalosis | • Respiratory acidosis |

## 7.9. Evaluation of Liver Function Tests

| Enzyme | Source | Increased | Decreased | Comments |
|---|---|---|---|---|
| 1. AST/ALT | • Liver<br>• Heart<br>• Skeletal muscle<br>• Pancreas<br>• RBCs<br>• Kidney | • Hepatocellular injury<br>• Rhabdomy-olysis<br>• Muscle dystrophy<br>• Hemolysis<br>• Liver cancer | • Vitamin $B_6$ deficiency<br>• Uremia | • ALT more specific than AST for liver<br>• AST>ALT in hemolysis<br>• AST/ALT > 2 in 90% of alcohol disorders in adults |
| 2. Alkaline phosphatase | • Liver<br>• Osteo-blasts<br>• Small intestine<br>• Kidney<br>• Placenta | • Hepatocellular injury<br>• Bone growth, disease, trauma<br>• Pregnancy<br>• Familial | • Low phosphate<br>• Wilson disease<br>• Zinc deficiency<br>• Hypothyroid-ism<br>• Pernicious anemia | • Highest in cholestatic conditions<br>• Must be dif-ferentiated from bone source |

*Contd...*

*Contd...*

| Enzyme | Source | Increased | Decreased | Comments |
|---|---|---|---|---|
| 3. GGT | • Bile ducts<br>• Renal tubules<br>• Pancreas<br>• Small intestine<br>• Brain | • Cholestasis<br>• Newborn period<br>• Induced by drugs | • Estrogen therapy<br>• Artificially low in hyperbilirubinemia | • Not found in bone<br>• Increased in 90% of primary liver disease<br>• Biliary obstruction<br>• Intrahepatic cholestasis<br>• Induced by alcohol<br>• Specific for hepatobiliary disease in nonpregnant patient |

## 7.10. Clues for Diagnosis of Functional Abdominal Pain

- Pain occurs longer than 3 months.
- Age of onset between 6 and 14 years of age.
- Child exhibits features of abdominal pain (grimacing, guarding abdominal muscles and rubbing painful areas).
- Physical and psychological stressors exacerbate the pain.
- Normal physical examination with no significant weight loss.
- Stool occult blood is negative.
- Normal laboratory testing (CBC, ESR, U/A, stool ova and parasites).

## 7.11. Clues that Indicate an Organic Cause for the Abdominal Pain

- Pain awakens the child at night
- Pain is localized or persistent away from umbilicus
- Weight loss or FTT
- Fever, rash, joint pain, mucous membrane changes/ulcers, dysuria
- Sleepiness following painful attacks
- Guaiac-positive stools
- Anemia
- Elevated ESR
- Family history of peptic ulcer disease or inflammatory bowel disease.

## 7.12. Holliday-Segar Formula

### 7.12.1. Holliday-Segar formula for daily calories required under basal conditions

- 100 kcal/kg for the first 10 kg plus
- 50 kcal/kg for the next 10 kg plus
- 20 kcal/kg for the rest of the weight.

### 7.12.2. Holliday-Segar formula for maintenance of calories and fluids

| Weight | kcal/day or mL/day | kcal/hour or mL/hour |
|---|---|---|
| 0–10 kg | 100/kg/day | 4/kg/hour |
| 11–20 kg | 1,000 + 50/kg/day* | 40 + 2/kg/hour |
| >20 kg | 1,500 + 20/kg/day** | 60 + 1/kg/hour** |
| * for each kg>10 | ** for each kg>20 | |

## 7.13. Foreign Body Ingestions

- Once in the stomach, nearly 95% of the foreign bodies will pass without problem.
- Diagnosis mostly can be with standard chest X-ray, because nearly 90% are radiopaque.
- Coins have a tendency to lie in the coronal plane (face forward) in the esophagus and the sagittal plane (on edge) in the trachea.

## 7.14. Certain Contraindications to Oral Replacement Therapy

- Shock
- Stool output > 10 mL/kg/hour
- Ileus
- Monosaccharide intolerance.

## 7.15. The "Rule of 2's" for Meckel Diverticulum

- Occurs in 2% of the population
- Localized within 2 feet of the ileocecal junction
- Measures 2 inches in length
- Measures 2 centimeters in diameter
- Male: female ratio is 2:1
- Usually symptomatic before 2 years of age.

## 7.16. Comparison of Ulcerative Colitis and Crohn Disease

|  | Ulcerative colitis (UC) | Crohn disease (CD) |
| --- | --- | --- |
| **Weight loss** | Some | Severe |
| **Growth failure** | Rare | Common |
| **Gross rectal bleeding** | Common | Less common |
| **Aphthous mouth ulcers** | Rare | Common |
| **Perianal lesions** | None | Common |
| **Bowel involvement** | Colon and rectum only | Anywhere from mouth to anus |
| **Pattern of lesions** | Continuous | Skip lesions |
| **Involvement of tissue** | Mucosal only | Transmural disease |
| **X-ray findings** | Superficial disease, loss of haustrations | Thumb printing, skip areas, string signs |
| **Granulomas likely** | No | Yes |
| **pANCA*** | 60% | 10–15% (mainly UC-like presentations) |
| **Anti-saccharomyces antibodies** | 5% | 60% |

*Antineutrophil cytoplasmic antibody staining with perinuclear highlighting

## 7.17. Who is at High-risk for Hepatitis A Infection or Complications

- High-risk behavior
- Children > 2 years old living in communities with high rates
- Chronic liver disease
- Travel to high-risk countries
- Patients with hepatitis B or C.

### 7.17.1. Hepatitis A; typical sequence of events following infection

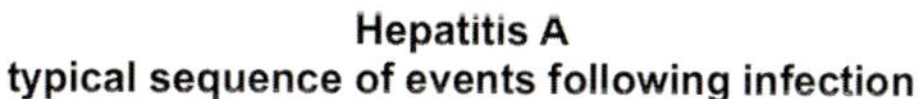
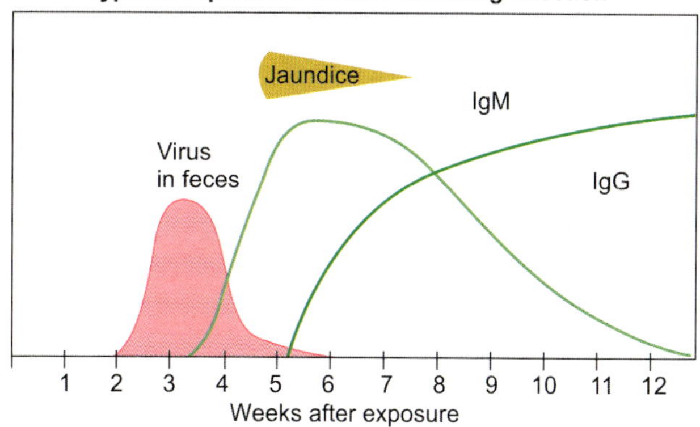


**Fig. 7.3**: Hepatitis A typical sequence of events

## 7.18. Hepatitis B (HBV)

### 7.18.1. The main 3 antigenic markers in hepatitis B

1.  HBsAg
2.  HBcAg
3.  HBeAg.

#### 7.18.1.1. Anti-HBs IgG

Finding anti-HBs IgG in the serum indicates:
• Past exposure to either hepatitis B virion or the vaccine
• Immunity to the virus.

#### 7.18.1.2. Anti-HBc IgG

The presence of anti-HBc IgG is the best marker for previous exposure to HBV.

#### 7.18.1.3. Anti-HBe IgG

The HBe antibodies appears several weeks after illness.

## 7.19.    Acute Hepatitis B Virus Infection with Recovery; Typical Serology Course

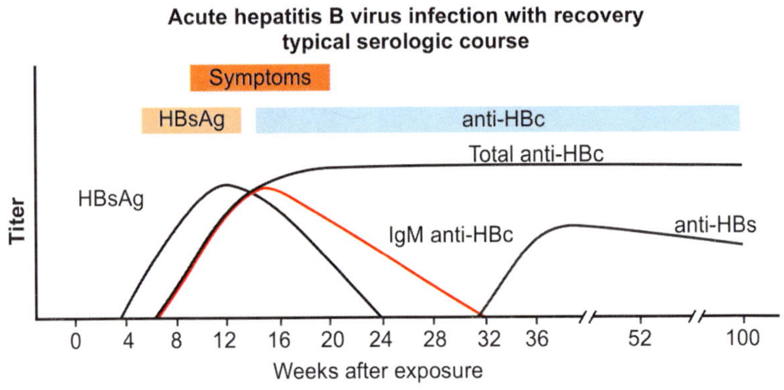

**Fig. 7.4**: Hepatitis B typical serology course

## 7.20.  The Rising and Falling Hepatitis B Serologic Markers after Months of Exposure

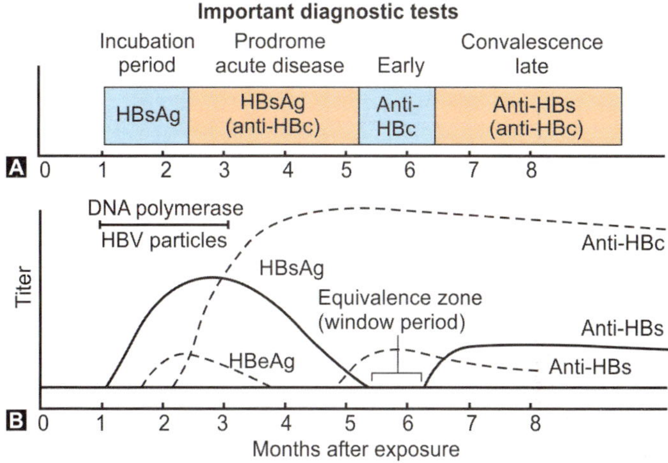



**Figs 7.5A and B**: Hepatitis B, important diagnostic tests. A: In acute infection and B: In chronic infection

## 7.21. The 3 Types of Carrier States Concerning Hepatitis B

1. Asymptomatic
2. Chronic persistent hepatitis
3. Chronic hepatitis B(CAH).

## 7.22. Possible Outcomes after Hepatitis B Infection

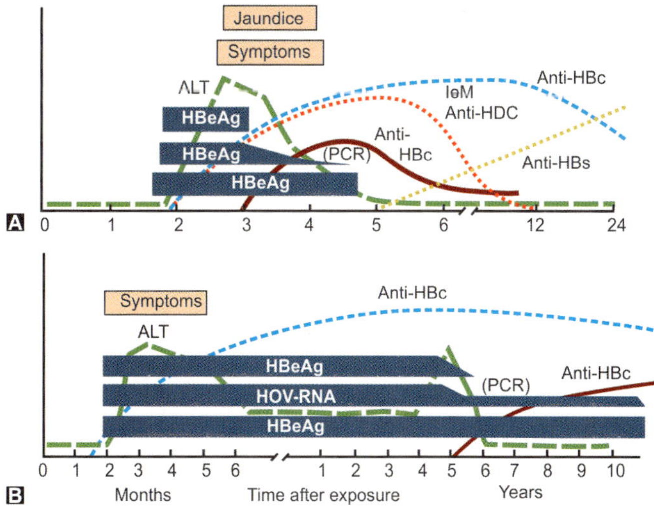



**Figs 7.6A and B**: Hepatitis B, possible outcomes. A: Acute infection and B: Chronic infection

## 7.23. Hepatitis B Scenarios

| HBsAg | HBcAb | HBsAb | Interpretation |
|---|---|---|---|
| + | - | - | Acute infection |
| + | + | - | 3-possibilities:<br>1. Acute infection<br>2. Chronic hepatitis B (high AST)<br>3. Carrier (normal enzymes) |
| - | - | + | 2- possibilities:<br>1. Remote infection<br>2. Immunized |
| - | + | + | Remote infection |
| - | + | - | 3-possibilities;<br>1. Window disease<br>2. Remote infection<br>3. False-positive |
| + | + | + | More than 1 infection, e.g. IV drug user or renal dialysis patient with both acute and chronic hepatitis B |

## 7.24. Types of Viral Hepatitis and their Serological Tests

| | Anti-HAV IgM | Anti-HAV IgG | HBsAg | Anti-HBs IgM | Anti-HBs IgG | Anti-HBc IgM | Anti-HBc IgG | HBeAg | Anti-HDV |
|---|---|---|---|---|---|---|---|---|---|
| Acute hepatitis A | + | - | | | | - | | | |
| Previous HAV | - | + | | | | - | | | |
| Acute HBV | - | | + Early | + Late | - | + | - | - | - |
| Acute HBV-window | | | - | - | - | + | - | - | - |
| Chronic active HBV | | | 95% | - | Rarely | - | + | Usually + | - |
| Remote HBV | | | - | - | + | - | + | - | - |
| Immunized –HBV | | | - | - | + | - | - | - | - |
| Acute hepatitis D-(with acute HBV) Early | | | + Early | + Late | - | + | - | + | + |
| Acute Hepatitis D-(with CAH) | | | 15% | - | Rarely | - | + | Usually + | + |

## 7.25. Conditions Associated with an Increased Risk of Hepatitis C

- IV drug abusers.
- Prisoners.
- High-risk sexual behavior: STDs, prostitutes, > 5 sexual partners a year.
- Blood transfusion before 1990.
- Tattoos and body piercing.
- Snoring cocaine.

## 7.26. Hepatitis E

- Unlike hepatitis A, hepatitis E carries a very high-risk for fulminant hepatitis in the third trimester of pregnancy—with a 20% fatality rate.
- With acute hepatitis and negative serology in a traveler think of hepatitis E.

## 7.27. Esophageal Atresia and Tracheoesophageal Fistula

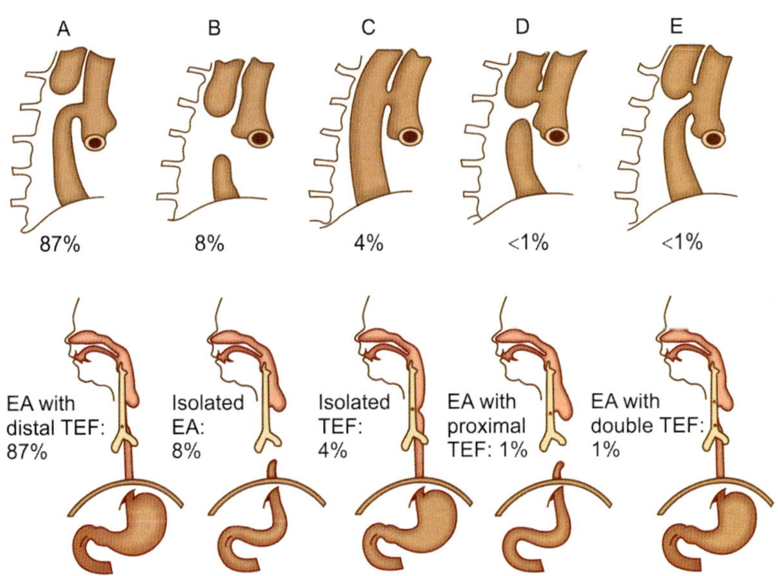


**Fig. 7.7**: Esophageal atresia and tracheoesophageal fistula

## 7.28. Types of Esophageal Hiatal Hernia

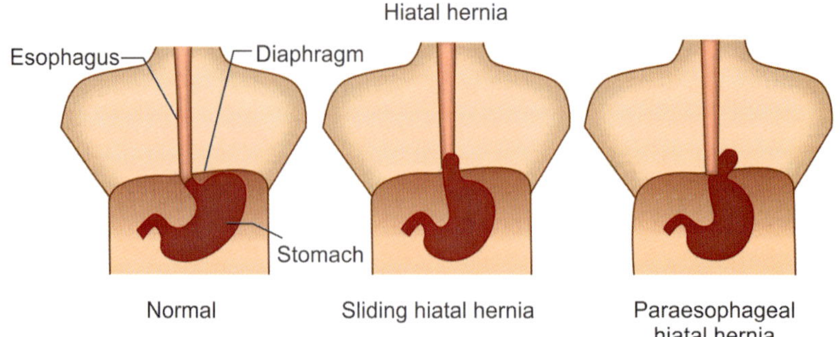


A. Sliding hiatal hernia (the most common type). B. Paraesophageal hiatal hernia

**Fig. 7.8**: Types of esophageal hiatal hernia

## 7.29. Congenital Duodenal Atresia

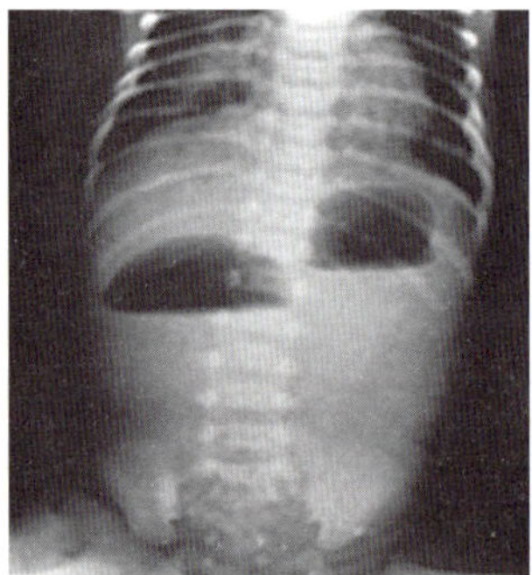

Abdominal radiograph of a newborn infant held upright. The "double-bubble" gas shadow above and the absence of gas in the distal bowel in this case of congenital duodenal atresia

**Fig. 7.9**: Radiograph of congenital duodenal atresia

## 7.30. Hypertrophic Pyloric Stenosis

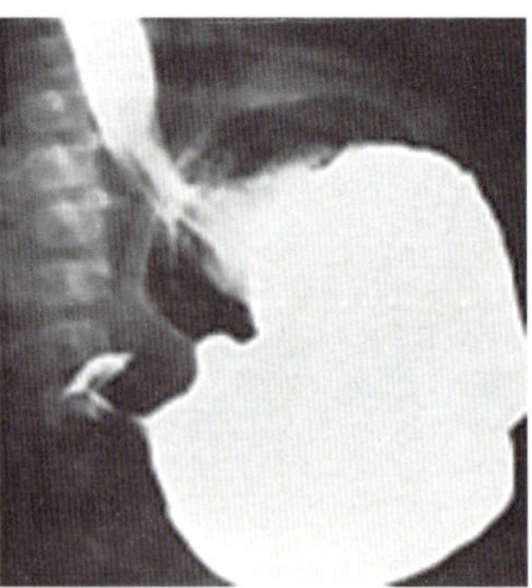

Barium in the stomach of an infant with projectile vomiting. The attenuated pyloric canal is typical of congenital hypertrophic pyloric stenosis

**Fig. 7.10**: Radiograph of hypertrophic pyloric stenosis

## 7.31. Most Common Causes of Oropharyngeal Dysphagia (Transfer Dysphagia)

Oropharyngeal dysphagia occurs when the transfer of the food bolus from the mouth to the esophagus is impaired.

1. Cerebral palsy
2. Cerebrovascular accidents
3. Myasthenia gravis
4. Botulism
5. Diphtheria
6. Inflammatory: Abscess and pharyngitis
7. Congenital web
8. Plummer-Vinson syndrome
9. Corrosive injury.

## 7.32. Most Common Causes of Esophageal Dysphagia

Esophageal dysphagia (difficulty in swallowing) occurs when there is difficulty in transporting the food bolus down the esophagus.

1. GERD
2. Foreign body
3. Esophagitis
4. Stricture: Corrosive injury and pill induced.

## 7.33. Common Causes of Emesis

### 7.33.1. Common causes of emesis during Infancy

1. Gastroenteritis
2. Gastroesophageal reflux
3. Overfeeding
4. Anatomic obstruction
   (Malrotation, pyloric stenosis and intussusception)
5. Systemic infection
6. Pertussis syndrome
7. Otitis media.

### 7.33.2. Common causes of emesis during childhood

1. Gastroenteritis
2. Systemic infection
3. Gastritis
4. Toxic ingestion
5. Pertussis syndrome
6. Medication

7. Reflux (GERD)
8. Sinusitis
9. Otitis media
10. Anatomic obstruction (malrotation and intussusception).

### 7.33.3. Common causes of emesis during adolescence

1. Gastroenteritis
2. GERD
3. Systemic infection
4. Toxic ingestion
5. Gastritis
6. Sinusitis
7. Inflammatory bowel disease
8. Appendicitis
9. Migraine
10. Pregnancy
11. Medication
12. Ipecac abuse and bulimia
13. Concussion.

## 7.34. Common Causes of Gastrointestinal Obstruction

### 7.34.1. Common congenital causes of intestinal obstruction

1. Esophageal atresia
2. Meconium ileus
3. Vascular rings
4. Meckel diverticulum with volvulus or intussusception
5. Pyloric stenosis
6. Meconium plug
7. Duodenal atresia
8. Hirschsprung disease
9. Malrotation/volvulus of small intestine
10. Imperforate anus
11. Malrotation/Ladd bands
12. Volvulus.

## 7.34.2. Common acquired causes of intestinal obstruction

1. Esophageal stricture
2. Foreign body
3. Achalasia
4. Bezoar and foreign body
5. Pyloric stricture (ulcer)
6. Postsurgical adhesions of small intestine
7. Intussusception
8. Ulcerative colitis (toxic megacolon).

## 7.35. Criteria for Cyclic Vomiting Syndrome

All of the criteria must be met for the consensus definition of cyclical vomiting syndrome:

1. At least 5 attacks in any interval, or a minimum of 3 attacks during a 6-month period.
2. Episodic attacks of intense nausea and vomiting lasting 1 hour to 10 days and occurring at least 1 week apart.
3. Stereotypical pattern and symptoms in the individual patient.
4. Vomiting during attacks occurs ≥4 times/hour for ≥1 hour.
5. Return to baseline health between episodes.
6. Not attributed to another disorder.

## 7.36. Complications of Vomiting

1. Metabolic: Alkalosis and hypochloremia
2. Nutritional
3. Mallory-Weiss tear
4. Esophagitis
5. Aspiration
6. Shock
7. Pneumomediastinum and pneumothorax
8. Petechiae and retinal hemorrhages.

## 7.37. Common Causes of Childhood Diarrhea

### 7.37.1. Common causes of acute childhood diarrhea

#### 7.37.1.1. Common causes of acute diarrhea in infancy

1. Gastroenteritis (viral > bacterial)
2. Systemic infection
3. Antibiotic associated
4. Overfeeding.

### 7.37.1.2. Common causes of acute diarrhea in children

1. Gastroenteritis (viral > bacterial)
2. Food poisoning
3. Systemic infection
4. Antibiotic associated.

### 7.37.1.3. Common causes of acute diarrhea in adolescence

1. Gastroenteritis (viral > bacterial)
2. Food poisoning
3. Antibiotic associated.

## 7.37.2. Common causes of chronic childhood diarrhea

### 7.37.2.1. Common causes of chronic diarrhea in infancy

1. Postinfectious secondary lactase deficiency
2. Cow's milk or soy protein intolerance
3. Chronic nonspecific diarrhea of infancy
4. Excessive fruit juice (sorbitol) ingestion
5. Celiac disease
6. Cystic fibrosis
7. AIDS enteropathy.

### 7.37.2.2. Common causes of chronic diarrhea in children

1. Postinfectious secondary lactase deficiency
2. Irritable bowel syndrome
3. Celiac disease
4. Lactose intolerance
5. Excessive fruit juice (sorbitol) ingestion
6. Giardiasis
7. Inflammatory bowel disease
8. AIDS enteropathy.

### 7.37.2.3. Common causes of chronic diarrhea in adolescence

1. Irritable bowel syndrome
2. Inflammatory bowel disease
3. Lactose intolerance
4. Giardiasis
5. Laxative abuse (anorexia nervosa)
6. Constipation with encopresis.

## 7.38. Common Causes of Constipation

- Nonorganic (functional)—Retentive
- Organic:
  1. Anal stenosis
  2. Anal stricture
  3. Hirschsprung disease
  4. Anticholinergics
  5. Hypothyroidism
  6. Diabetes mellitus and diabetes insipidus
  7. Anorexia nervosa.

## 7.39. Chronic Abdominal Pain in Children

### 7.39.1. Nonorganic causes of chronic abdominal pain

1. Functional abdominal pain
2. Irritable bowel syndrome
3. Nonulcer dyspepsia.

### 7.39.2. Gastrointestinal tract causes of chronic abdominal pain

1. Chronic constipation
2. Lactose intolerance
3. Parasite infection (specially *Giardia*)
4. Excess fructose or sorbitol ingestion
5. Crohn disease
6. Peptic ulcer
7. Esophagitis
8. Meckel's diverticulum
9. Recurrent intussusception
10. Chronic appendicitis or appendiceal mucocele.

### 7.39.3. Gallbladder and pancreas tract causes of chronic abdominal pain

1. Cholelithiasis
2. Choledochal cyst
3. Recurrent pancreatitis.

### 7.39.4. Genitourinary tract causes of chronic abdominal pain

1. Urinary tract infection
2. Hydronephrosis
3. Urolithiasis.

### 7.39.5. Miscellaneous causes of chronic abdominal pain

1. Abdominal migraine
2. Abdominal epilepsy
3. Gilbert syndrome
4. Familial mediterranean fever
5. Sickle cell crisis
6. Lead poisoning
7. Henoch-Schönlein purpura
8. Angioneurotic edema
9. Acute intermittent porphyria.

## 7.40. Common Causes of Gastrointestinal Bleeding in Childhood

### 7.40.1. Common causes of gastrointestinal bleeding in infancy

1. Bacterial enteritis
2. Milk protein allergy
3. Intussusception
4. Swallowed maternal blood
5. Anal fissure
6. Lymphonodular hyperplasia.

### 7.40.2. Common causes of gastrointestinal bleeding in children

1. Bacterial enteritis
2. Anal fissure
3. Colonic polyps
4. Intussusception
5. Peptic ulcer/gastritis
6. Swallowed epistaxis
7. Prolapse (traumatic) gastropathy secondary to emesis
8. Mallory-Weiss syndrome.

### 7.40.3. Common causes of gastrointestinal bleeding in adolescence

1. Bacterial enteritis
2. Inflammatory bowel disease
3. Peptic ulcer/gastritis
4. Prolapse (traumatic) gastropathy secondary to emesis
5. Mallory-Weiss syndrome
6. Colonic polyps
7. Anal fissure.

## Bibliography


1. emedicalppt.blogspot.com
2. http://emedicine.medscape.com
3. http://www.asha.org/public/speech/swallowing/feedswallowchildren.htm
4. http://www.cdc.gov/hepatitis
5. http://www.cmnb.org
6. http://www.ncbi.nlm.nih.gov/pmc/articles/PMC2904303/
7. http://www.webmd.com/digestive-disorders/cyclic-vomiting-syndrome



## Bibliography

1. emedicalppt.blogspot.com
2. http://emedicine.medscape.com
3. http://www.asha.org/public/speech/swallowing/feedswallowchildren.htm
4. http://www.cdc.gov/hepatitis
5. http://www.cmnb.org

## 8.1. Indications for Genetic Counseling

| | |
|---|---|
| Advanced parental age:<br>• Maternal age ≥35 years | • Paternal age ≥50 years |
| Previous child with or family history of:<br>• Congenital abnormality<br>• Dysmorphology<br>• Mental retardation<br>• Isolated birth defect | • Metabolic disorder<br>• Chromosome abnormality<br>• Single-gene disorder |
| Consanguinity | Teratogen exposure (occupational and abuse) |
| Repeated pregnancy loss or infertility | |
| Pregnancy screening abnormality:<br>• Maternal serum α-fetoprotein<br>• Fetal ultrasonography<br>• Fetal karyotype | Heterozygote screening based on ethnic risk:<br>• Sickle cell anemia<br>• Tay-Sachs, Canavan, Gaucher diseases<br>• Thalassemias |

## 8.2. Pedigree Symbols

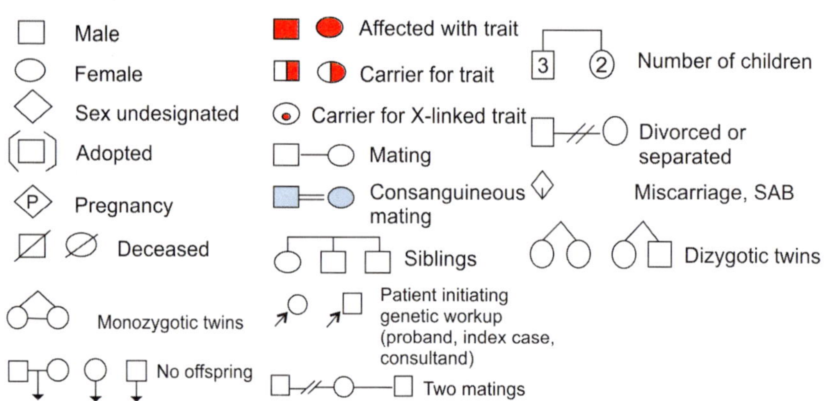


**Fig. 8.1**: Pedigree symbols

## 8.3. Autosomal Dominant (AD) Inheritance

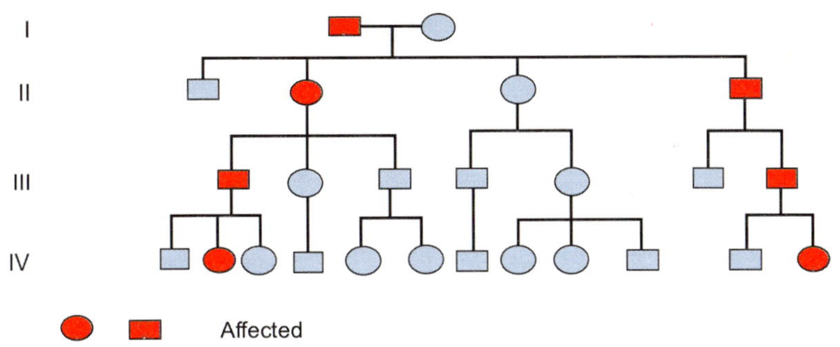



**Fig. 8.2**: Autosomal dominant inheritance

The above pedigree shows the followings:

- Both sexes are equally affected.
- Both sexes can transmit to offspring.
- No generation is skipped (unless the trait is subtle or not completely expressed then you may not notice it in that generation).
- Every affected child has a parent with the disorder (except if this is a new gene mutation; then this child's offspring will have a 50% risk of inheriting this gene mutation).
- There is father-to-child transmission (This excludes all X-linked and mitochondrial transmission).

## 8.4. Autosomal Recessive (AR) Inheritance

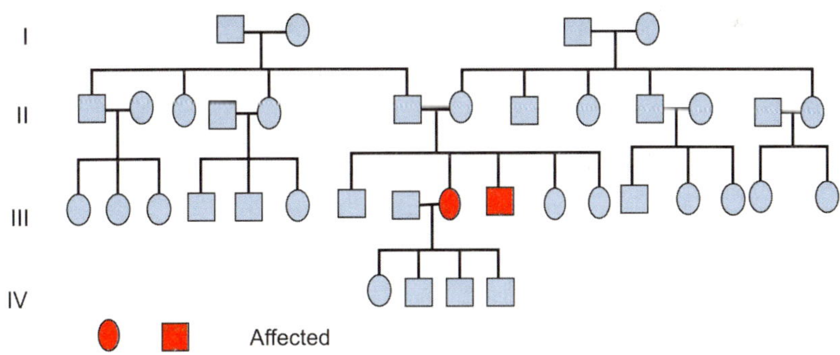



**Fig. 8.3**: Autosomal recessive inheritance

**The above pedigree shows the followings:**

- Both sexes are equally affected.
- Males and females can each transmit the altered allele.
- Disorder in one or more siblings but not in other generation.

- The risk for 2 heterozygotes to have an affected offspring is ¼ (2 heterozygote also can have offspring who are all affected or all unaffected).
- Consanguinity increases the risk of having an offspring with an AR disorder (figure below)

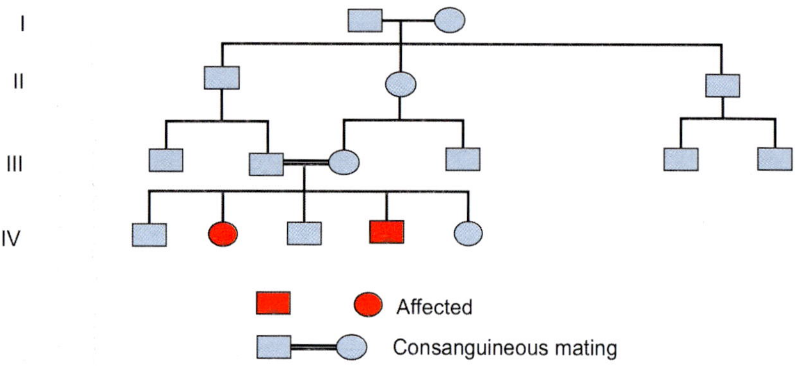



**Fig. 8.4**: Autosomal recessive shows consanguineous mating

## 8.5. X-linked Recessive (XR) Inheritance

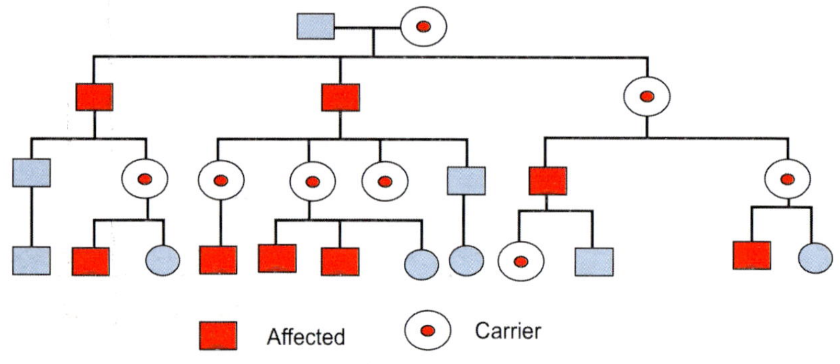



**Fig. 8.5**: Sex-linked recessive inheritance

**The above pedigree shows the followings:**
- Only females can transmit the disease to their sons, there is never male-to-male transmission.
- If a generation has only females, the disease will appear to have "Skipped" that generation.
- An affected father transmits the disease allele to all his daughters (the daughters are obligate carriers, but usually unaffected).
- Carrier females have a 50% chance of transmitting the disease to their sons.

## 8.6. Y-linked Inheritance

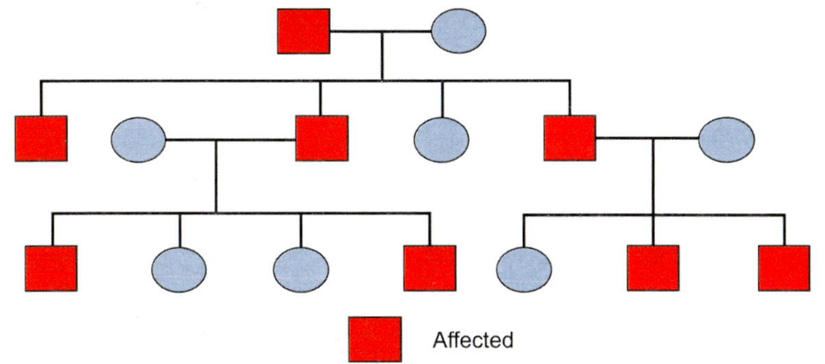



**Fig. 8.6**: Y-linked inheritance

- Only male-to-male transmission.
- Only males are affected.
- Most Y-linked genes are related to male sex determination and reproduction and are associated with infertility.
- It is rare to see familial transmission of a Y-linked disorder.
- Leri-Weil dyschondrosteosis:
  - A rare skeletal dysplasia that involves bilateral bowing of the forearms with dislocations of the ulna at the wrist and generalized short stature.
  - It is a heterozygous mutations on Y-chromosome.

## 8.7. Mitochondrial Inheritance

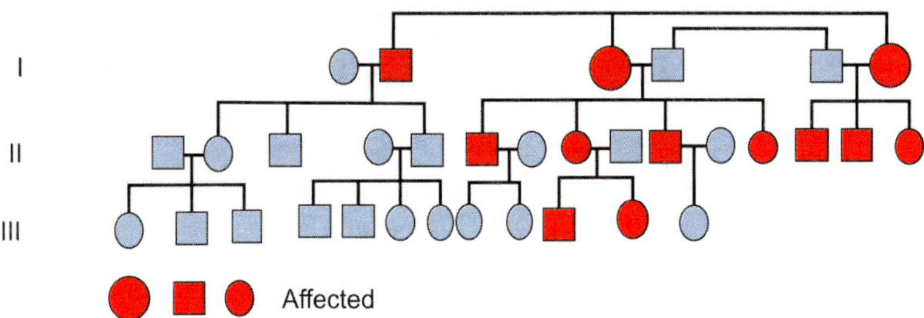



**Fig. 8.7**: Mitochondrial inheritance

The above pedigree shows the followings:
- Mitochondrial inheritance is unique because the ovum, not the sperm, transmits all the mitochondria to their zygote.
- A mother carrying a mitochondrial DNA (m-DNA) mutation will pass it on to all her offspring.
- The father carrying the mutation passes it to none.

Few disorders that are caused by mutations in the mitochondrial genome.

### 8.7.1. Myoclonic epilepsy and red-ragged fibers (MERRF)

- Progressive myoclonic epilepsy
- Myopathy
- Dementia
- Hearing loss.

### 8.7.2.  Mitochondrial encephalopathy, with stroke-like episodes, and lactic acidosis (MELAS)

MELAS present anytime between the ages of toddler and adolescent.

### 8.7.3. Leigh disease

- Basal ganglia defects
- Hypotonia
- Optic atrophy.

In infancy and early childhood.

### 8.7.4. Kearns-Sayre syndrome

- Ophthalmoplegia
- Retinitis pigmentosa
- Myopathy
- Cardiac conduction defects
- Pearson syndrome
- Anemia
- Neutropenia
- Pancreatic dysfunction
- Myopathy in infants.

## 8.8.  Clues that Genetic Disorder is likely

- Previous family history of genetic disorder
- Positive neonatal screen
- Congenital anomalies
- Developmental abnormalities
- Neurologic disorders
- Death in utero or soon after birth
- Growth abnormalities
- Multiorgan dysfunction.

## 8.9. Indications for Chromosomal Analysis

- Multiple birth defects
- Developmental delay and/or mental retardation
- Growth abnormalities (e.g. short stature)
- Abnormal sexual development
- Recurrent miscarriages.

## 8.10.  Abnormal Maternal Screen Study

The followings are indicators of increase risk of a fetus with Down syndrome during serum screening of women under 35 years of age.
- Low maternal serum $\alpha$-fetoprotein
- Low unconjugated estriol
- Elevated $\beta$-HCG [human chorionic gonadotropin]
- Elevated inhibin A.

## 8.11. Down Syndrome Features

### 8.11.1. Most commonly found in Down syndrome

- Hypotonia
- Small ears
- Mental retardation.

### 8.11.2. More specific to Down syndrome

- Brachydactyly
- Absent-to very-small nipple buds
- Central placement of the posterior hair whorl.

### 8.11.3. Common in Down syndrome, but nonspecific

- Microcephaly
- Up-slanted palpebral fissures
- Flat midface
- Full cheeks
- Epicanthal folds
- Single transverse crease
- Speckled irises (Brushfield spots)
- High-arched palate
- Hypoplasia of the middle phalanx of 5th finger/clinodactyly.

### 8.11.4. Ophthalmological features in Down syndrome

1.   Up-slanted palpebral fissures
2.   Blepharospasm
3.   Epicanthal folds
4.   Nystagmus
5.   Strabismus and refractory  errors (very common)
6.   Speckled irises (Brushfield spots)
7.   Eccentric pupils
8.   Cataracts (congenital in 5%).

### 8.11.5. Heart defects in Down syndrome

*   Heart defects are fairly common, occurring in nearly 50%.
*   1/3rd of these are AV canal defects.
*   1/3rd are VSDs.
*   1/3rd of them have ASDs of the secundum variety and tetralogy of Fallot.

### 8.11.6. Gastrointestinal defects in Down syndrome

*   Duodenal atresia and Hirschsprung disease occur in about 5% of infants.

### 8.11.7. Other problems of Down syndrome in childhood

*   Hypothyroidism
*   Atlantoaxial instability
*   Leukemia.

### 8.11.8. Problems of older patients with Down syndrome

*   DM
*   Thyroid disorders (both hypo and hyperthyroidism)
*   Atlantoaxial subluxation
*   Cataracts
*   Leukemia
*   Seizures
*   Cognitive dysfunction (during the 40s)
*   Dementia or early-onset Alzheimer disease.

### 8.11.9. Anticipatory guidance for children with Down syndrome

| Evaluation | Time of evaluation |
|---|---|
| All routine immunizations | |
| Cardiac evaluation with echocardiogram | Newborn period |
| Ophthalmologic evaluation | Before 6 months of age |
| Hearing evaluation | By 6 months of age |
| Newborn screening for hypothyroidism | Do thyroid function studies (T4, TSH) at 3, 6, and 12 months and then annually |
| Vision screening | At age 4 years |
| Order C-spine X-rays | At ~ 3 years of age, to monitor for atlantoaxial instability |

### 8.11.10. Associated findings with Down syndrome

| Associated findings | Percentage |
|---|---|
| Mental retardation | 100% |
| Hearing loss | 66% |
| Eye disease | 60% |
| Serous otitis media | 60%–80% |
| Cardiac defects | 40% |
| Thyroid disease | 15% |
| Gastrointestinal atresias | 12% |
| Atlantoaxial instability | 12%–20% |
| Leukemia | 1% |

## 8.12.  Characteristic Findings of Trisomy 18 (Edwards' Syndrome)

- Intrauterine growth restriction.
- High forehead.
- Small face and mouth.
- Rocker bottom feet.
- Overlapping fingers.
- Structural heart defects (90%); most often a VSD with multiple dysplastic valves.
- 40% dying by 1 year of age (most die due to central apnea).
- Mental retardation.
- Microcephaly.

- Short sternum.
- Clubfoot /clinched fist.
- Hypoplastic nails.
- 50% of affected children die in the 1st week of life.
- Those who survive past 1 year of age typically function on a 6–12-month-old level.

### 8.13. Common Clinical Findings of Trisomy 13 (Patau Syndrome) (Think of Midline Defects)

- Orofacial cleft
- Microphthalmia
- Postaxial polydactyly of the limbs
- Holoprosencephaly
- Heart malformations (80%)
- Hypoplastic or absent ribs
- Genital anomalies
- Abdominal wall defects
- Cutis aplasia.

### 8.14. Turner Syndrome—45, X

#### 8.14.1. Common clinical findings of Turner syndrome—45, X

- Short female with broad chest
- Wide-spaced nipples
- Webbed neck
- Congenital lymphedema
- Pubertal delay
- Left-sided heart defects.

#### 8.14.2. Associated findings with Turner syndrome—45, X

| Associated findings | Percentage |
| --- | --- |
| Gonadal dysgenesis | 90% |
| Renal anomalies | 60% |
| Hearing loss | 50% |
| Cardiac defects | 10%–30% |

## 8.15. Common Clinical Findings of Fragile X Syndrome

| | |
|---|---|
| Boys: | Prevalence: 1 in 1,250–2,500 males<br>Phenotype most prominent in boys |

- Mild to profound mental retardation
- Cluttered speech
- Autism (60%)
- Macrocephaly
- Large ears
- Prognathism
- Postpubertal macro-orchidism
- Tall stature

| | |
|---|---|
| Girls: | Prevalence: 1 in 1,600–5,000 females<br>May have only  learning disabilities |

## 8.16. Common Clinical Findings of Klinefelter Syndrome—47, XXY

Prevalence: 1 in 500 males

- Mean full scale IQ 85–90
- Behavior problems
- Low upper to lower body ratio
- Small testes
- Inadequate testosterone production
- Infertility
- Gynecomastia
- Increased risk of extragonadal germ cell tumors.

## 8.17. Indications for Karyotype

1. Two major or one major and two minor malformations (include: small for gestational age and mental retardation as major).
2. Features of a specific chromosomal syndrome.
3. At risk for familial chromosomal aberration.
4. Ambiguous genitalia.
5. More than two spontaneous abortions or infertility (karyotype both partners).
6. Girls with short stature.

## Bibliography


1. http://110.164.68.234/infotech/files/Genetics
2. http://ghr.nlm.nih.gov/handbook/inheritance/inheritancepatterns
3. http://hihg.med.miami.edu
4. http://www.geneticseducation.nhs.uk/genetics-glossary/212-mitochondrial-inheritance
5. http://www.nhs.uk/Conditions/Downs-syndrome/Pages/Symptoms.aspx
6. https://migrc.org/Library/Ylinked.html

# Growth and Development

## 9.1. Predicting Midparental Height in Children

Midparental height in girls:

$$\frac{(\text{father's height} - 13 \text{ cm}) + (\text{mother's height})}{2}$$

Midparental height in boys:

$$\frac{(\text{mother's height} + 13 \text{ cm}) + (\text{father's height})}{2}$$

## 9.2. Quick Pearls to Remember about Growth

### 9.2.1. Birth weight

- Regained by 10–14 days of life
- Doubles by 4 months
- Triples by 12 months
- Quadruples by 24 months.

After 2 years of age, normal weight gain is 5 lb/year until adolescence.

### 9.2.2. Birth length

- Increases by 50% at 1 year
- Doubles by 4 years
- Triples by 13 years.

After 2 years of age, average height increase is 2″/year until adolescence.

### 9.2.3. Head growth

The largest rate of growth is between 0 and 2 months (0.5 cm/week).

## 9.3. Definitions of Failure to Thrive (FTT)

### 9.3.1. One point on the growth curve

Weight:
- <3rd percentile

- For height <5th percentile
- 20% or more below ideal weight for height.

### 9.3.2. A series of points on the growth curve

Weight:
- Gain <20 gm/day from 0–3 months of age
- Gain <15 gm/day from 3–6 months of age
- Downward crossing of ≥ 2 major percentiles.

## 9.4. Developmental Milestones

### 9.4.1. Reflexes

| | |
|---|---|
| Moro | Absent by 3–4 months |
| Palmar grasp | Absent by 2–3 months |
| Parachute | Present by 6–9 months |

### 9.4.2. Head control

| When lying down: | |
|---|---|
| Lifts head momentarily | 1 month |
| Head upto 45 degrees | 2 months |
| Head upto 90 degrees | 3–4 months |
| **When pull to sitting:** | |
| Complete head lag | Newborn |
| No head lag | 5 months |
| Lifts head off table in anticipation of being lifted | 6 months |

### 9.4.3. Rolling and sitting

| Rolling: | |
|---|---|
| Rolls front to back | 4–5 months |
| Rolls back to front | 5–6 months |
| **Sitting:** | |
| Sits without support | 7 months |

### 9.4.4. Hands/Fingers

| | |
|---|---|
| Voluntary grasp (no release) | 5 months |
| Transfers objects between hands | 6 months |
| Uses thumb to grasp cube | 6–8 months |
| "Mature" cube grasp (finger and distal thumb) | 10–12 months |
| Plays "pat-a-cake" | 9–10 months |
| Tower of 2 cubes | 13–15 months |
| Tower of 4 cubes | 18 months |
| Uses cup and spoon well | 15–18 months |

### 9.4.5. Ambulating

| **Walking:** | |
|---|---|
| Pulls to stand | 9 months |
| Walks holding onto furniture | 11 months |
| Walks without help | 13 months |
| Walks well | 15 months |
| Runs well | 2 years |
| **Stairs:** | |
| Up and downstairs, 2 feet each step | 2 years |
| Up and downstairs, 1 foot per step each way | 4 years |
| **Jumps:** | |
| Jumps off ground with 2 feet up | 2.5 years |
| Hops on 1 foot | 4 years |
| Skips | 5–6 years |
| Balances on one foot 2–3 seconds | 3 years |
| Balances on one foot 6–10 seconds | 4 years |

### 9.4.6. Social

| | |
|---|---|
| Social smile | 1–2 months |
| Smiles at mirror | 5 months |
| Separation anxiety | 6–12 months |
| Waves "bye-bye" | 10 months |
| Dresses self (except buttons in back) | 2 years |
| Ties shoe laces | 5 years |
| Parallel play | 1–2 years |
| Cooperative play | 3–4 years |
| Can tell fantasy from reality | 5 years |

### 9.4.7. Speech and language

| | |
|---|---|
| Coos | 2–4 months |
| First words | 9–12 months |
| Understands 1-step commands | 15 months |
| Vocabulary of 10–15 words | 13–18 months |
| 2-words sentences | 18–24 months |
| 3-words sentences | 2–3 years |
| 4-words sentences | 3–4 years |

## 9.5. Tooth Development

| Teeth | Erupt | Fall out |
|---|---|---|
| Central incisors | 6–12 months | 6–10 years |
| Lateral incisors | 7–16 months | 7–8 years |
| Canines or cuspids | 16–23 months | 9–11 years |
| First molars | 12–19 months | 9–11 years |
| Second molars | 20–33 months | 10–12 years |

## 9.6. Routine Childhood Immunization Administration

### 9.6.1.

All routine childhood immunizations are IM (intramuscular) except for:
- 3 SubQ (subcutaneous):
  1. MMR
  2. Varicella
  3. IPV.
- 1 oral: Rotavirus.

### 9.6.2. Live vaccines include

1. MMR
2. Varicella
3. Rotavirus
4. OPV
5. Oral typhoid (rarely given, except for travel)
6. Yellow fever (rarely given, except for travel).

### 9.6.3. OPV

OPV is contraindicated in both an immunocompromised household and patient.

### 9.6.4. Anaphylactic reaction associated with special vaccines

If a patient has had an anaphylactic reaction to one of the following, perform skin testing to determine safety of the corresponding vaccine.

- Egg antigens: Influenza and yellow fever
- Streptomycin, neomycin, polymyxin B:IPV and OPV
- Neomycin: MMR and varicella
- Gelatin: MMR, varicella and yellow fever.

### 9.6.5. Facts about vaccination
#### 9.6.5.1.

There is no contraindication to vaccinating someone with severe egg allergy with MMR or its components.

#### 9.6.5.2.

Vaccinate those children with functional/anatomical asplenia (patients with sickle cell,  hemoglobinopathy or AIDS), with Hib vaccine, regardless of age (even > 5 years).

#### 9.6.5.3.

- If the mother is HBsAg+ or her status in unknown give hepatitis B vaccine at birth or within 12 hours.
- If mother is HBsAg+, also give HBIG (hepatitis B immune globin) within 12 hours of delivery at a different site.

### 9.7. Screening Scheme for Development Delay Upper Range

| Age (Month) | Gross motor | Fine motor | Social skills | Language |
| --- | --- | --- | --- | --- |
| 3 | Supports weight on forearms | Opens hands spontaneously | Smiles appropriately | Coos and laughs |
| 6 | Sits momentarily | Transfers objects | Shows likes and dislikes | Babbles |
| 9 | Pulls to stand | Pincer grasp | Play Pat-a-cake, Peek-a-boo | Initiates sounds |
| 12 | Walks with one hand held | Releases an object on command | Comes when called | 1–2 meaningful words |
| 18 | Walks upstairs with assistance | Feeds from a spoon | Mimics action of others | At least 6 words |
| 24 | Runs | Built  a tower of 6 blocks | Plays with others | 2–3 words sentence |

## 9.8. Expressive Language Development

| | |
|---|---|
| 6 months | • Babbles<br>• Different cries noted |
| 12 months | • Points<br>• Shakes head<br>• "Mama" or "Dada" |
| 18 months | • Uses gestures well<br>• Has about a 15–20 words vocabulary<br>• Uses 2–3 word phrases<br>• Speaks in a way that immediate household family members can understand |
| 24 months | • Expanding vocabulary<br>• More fluency-less stuttering<br>• About 25% of words are intelligible to strangers |
| 3 years | • Can use complete sentences<br>• Talks in short paragraphs<br>• Most words are intelligible to strangers<br>• Uses plurals, pronouns and prepositions |
| 4 years | • Can use past tense<br>• 4–5 word sentences<br>• Short paragraphs<br>• Able to tell a story or explain a recent event |

## 9.9. Clues to Abnormal Speech and Language Development by Age

| | |
|---|---|
| 12–15 months | Is not babbling or using different sounds |
| 18–24 months | Uses only a few words, hardly any phrase |
| 2 years | • Cannot follow simple directions<br>• Points instead of speaking<br>• Is not using 2-syllable words or combining words |
| 2½ years | • Cannot be understood most of the time<br>• Frequently omits first or last consonant of a word<br>• Cannot understand 2-step directions<br>• Cannot pronounce: b, h, m, n, p ,w |
| 3 years | Cannot repeat a 4- or 5-word sentence |
| 3½ years | • Cannot name specific objects easily<br>• Omits words in sentences<br>• Cannot pronounce: d, f, g, k, t |
| 4 years | Cannot tell a simple story |
| 5 years | Cannot pronounce :1, j, v, ch, sh |
| 6 years | Cannot pronounce: r, s, z, st, th |

## 9.10. Factors Associated with Hearing Loss in Neonates

1. Family history of sensorineural hearing loss.
2. Congenital infection.
3. Presence of craniofacial anomalies.
4. Birth weight is below 1,500 gm.
5. Neonatal jaundice resulting in exchange transfusion.
6. Ototoxic medications (furosemide and aminoglycosides).
7. Bacterial meningitis.
8. Apgar scores of 3 or less at 5 minutes.
9. Physical findings consistent with a syndrome  associated with hearing loss.

## 9.11. Behaviors Suggestive of ADHD

1. Inattentive behaviors
2. Easily distracted by  extraneous stimuli
3. Makes careless mistakes in school/work or other activities
4. Has difficulty maintaining attention to task
5. Does not seem to listen to what is being said to them
6. Fails to finish schoolwork and chores or other duties
7. Loses things necessary for tasks or activities
8. Has difficulty organizing tasks and activities
9. Forgetful in daily activities
10. Hyperactive/impulsive behaviors
11. Runs about or climbs excessively in inappropriate situation
12. Fidgets with hands or feet or squirms
13. Has difficulty awaiting turn in games or groups
14. Blurts out answers to questions.

## 9.12.  Suggested Metabolic Syndrome Indices in Children and Adolescents

1. BMI: >97th percentile
2. Triglycerides: >100 mg/dL
3. HDL cholesterol: <40 mg/dL
4. Systolic/diastolic BP: >90th percentile
5. Glucose abnormalities:
   - Fasting glucose >110 mg/dL  or
   - Oral glucose tolerance test >14 mg/dL.
6. Waist circumference: > 90th percentile.

## 9.13. Grasping and Handedness: Facts

1. Voluntary, accurate release is as essential as grasping for later manipulative skills.
2. Handedness (which hand is dominant) is clear in many children by 24 months and is expected in the majority by 42 months.
3. Delayed development of which hand is dominant is frequently associated with specific as well as general learning difficulties.

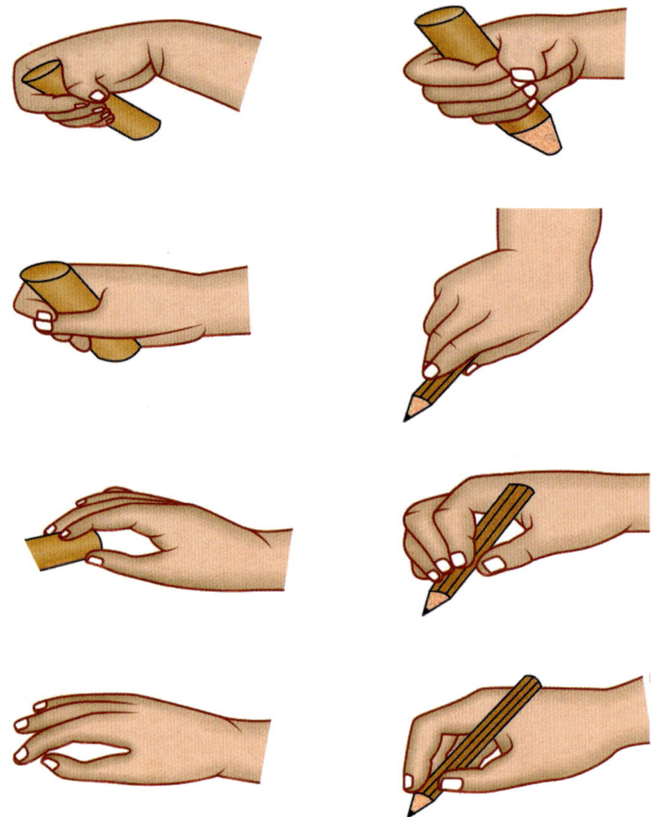

**Fig. 9.1**: Grasping and handedness

## 9.14. Social Learning, Self and Others, Play and Adaptive Skills Include

1. The child's social reactions to other persons and to peers through the development of attachments and social understanding.
2. Development of self-awareness and self-regulation.
3. Mastery of skills such as feeding, elimination and dressing.

## 9.15. Constructional and Drawing Skills

| Age | Block test | | Pencil test | |
|---|---|---|---|---|
| 3 – 3½ years | Build a bridge 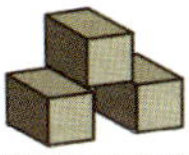 | | Draw a circle 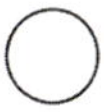 | |
| 3½ – 4 years | | | Draw a cross 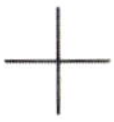 | |
| 3 – 4½ years | Build a gate 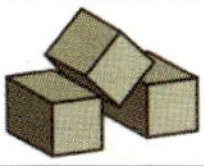 | | Draw a square 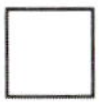 | |
| 5 – 6 years | Build steps 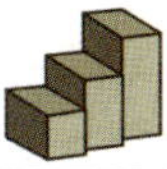 | | Draw a triangle 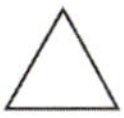 | |

**Fig. 9.2**: Constructional and drawing skills

## 9.16. Importance of Skill Delays

Delays in some areas of development are more important for long-term learning than others:

1. Developmental delay in motor skills only is of much less long-term significance than persistent significant delays in language and cognitive skills.
2. Self-help competence, for example toilet training, feeding and dressing, can also be dissociated from the level of general learning.
3. Some skills (e.g. symbolic play and language) reflect understanding of the environment and are therefore better indicators of intellectual ability.
4. Make allowance for prematurity less than 12 months.

## 9.17. The Differential Diagnosis of Delay in Motor Milestones

1. Normal variant, e.g. shuffler, roller, asymmetrical head turner, toe walker - ask about family history; shuffling and other patterns may have a genetic predisposition.
2. Global delay/general learning difficulties/mental retardation.
3. Cerebral palsy/other neurological disorder.
4. Early presentation of developmental coordination problems—Hypotonia and delay.
5. Connective tissue disorder.

## 9.18. Specific Neurodevelopmental Impairments Include

1. Specific developmental disorders of speech and language.
2. Specific developmental disorders of acquired academic skills, for example reading, spelling and mathematics.
3. Specific developmental disorders of motor function (developmental co-ordination disorder—Clumsy child).
4. Autistic spectrum disorders (also called the pervasive developmental disorders).
5. Specific impairments of memory (short or long-term episodic or declarative) and learning.
6. Specific developmental impairments of attention.
7. Specific developmental impairment of executive function.

## 9.19. Classification of Sexual Maturity States in Girls

| SMR stage | Pubic hair | Breast |
|---|---|---|
| 1 | Preadolescent | Preadolescent |
| 2 | Sparse, lightly pigmented, straight and medial border of labia | Breast and papilla elevated as small mound; diameter of areola increased |
| 3 | Darker, beginning to curl and increased amount | Breast and areola enlarged, no contour separation |
| 4 | Coarse, curly and abundant but less than in adult | Areola and papilla form secondary mound |
| 5 | Adult feminine triangle and spread to medial surface of thighs | Mature, nipple projects and areola part of general breast contour |

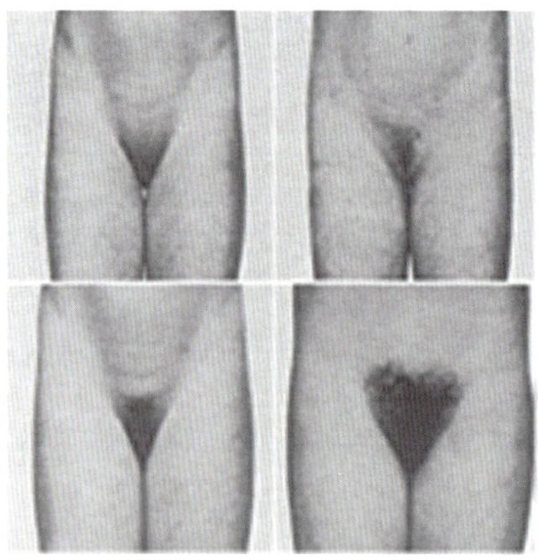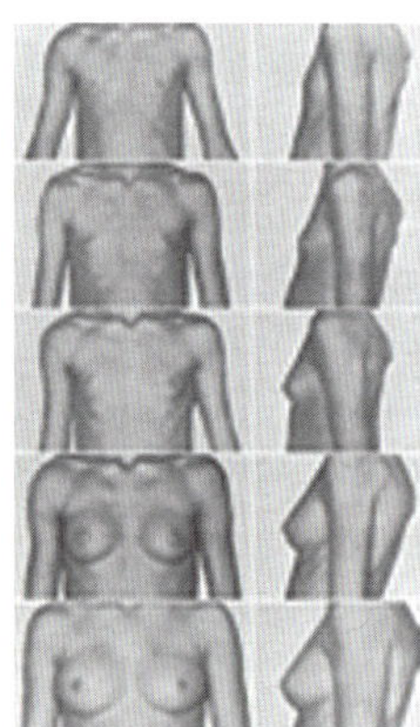

**Fig. 9.3**: SMR in girls

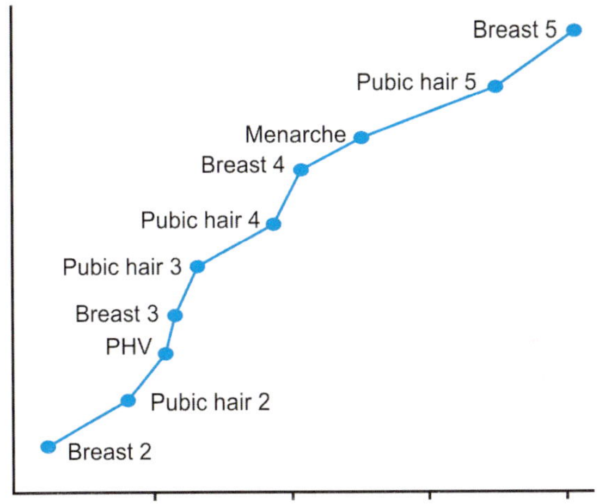



**Fig. 9.4**: Sequence of pubertal events in females

## 9.20. Classification of Sexual Maturity States in Boys

| SMR stage | Pubic hair | Penis | Testes |
|---|---|---|---|
| 1 | None | Preadolescent | Preadolescent |
| 2 | Scanty, long and slightly pigmented | Minimal change/ enlargement | Enlarged scrotum pink, and texture altered |
| 3 | Darker, starting to curl and small amount | Lengthens | Larger |
| 4 | Resembles adult type, but less quantity; coarse and curly | Larger; glans and breadth increase in size | Larger and scrotum dark |
| 5 | Adult distribution and spread to medial surface of thighs | Adult size | Adult size |

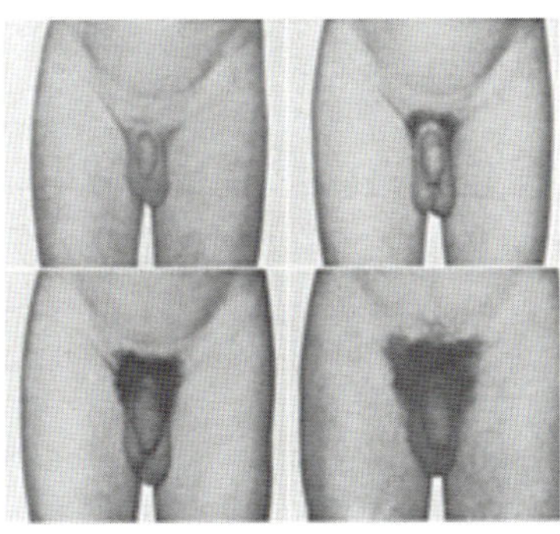

**Fig. 9.5**: SMR in boys

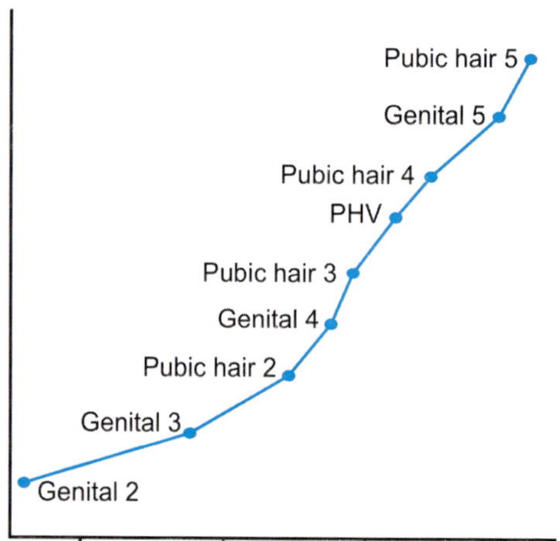


**Fig. 9.6**: Sequence of pubertal events in males

## Bibliography

1. http://www.aafp.org/afp/2011/0401/p829.html
2. http://www.cdc.gov/ncbddd/actearly/milestones/index.html
3. http://www.cdc.gov/vaccines/recs/vac-admin
4. http://www.med.umich.edu/1libr/pa/umsound_riskfactors.htm
5. http://www.speech-language-therapy.com
6. http://www.unicef.org/earlychildhood/files/Activity_Guide.pdf
7. http://www.who.int/ceh/capacity/neurodevelopmental.pdf
8. www.mja.com.au

## 10.1. Anemia Mechanism Summary

### 10.1.1. Proliferation defect (production)

| Reticulocyte count | Morphology | Etiology | Examples |
| --- | --- | --- | --- |
| Decreased | Normal | 1. Decreased erythropoietin<br>2. Bone marrow failure | 1. Chronic kidney disease<br>2. Aplastic anemia |

### 10.1.2. Maturation Defect

#### *10.1.2.1. Cytoplasmic maturation defect*

| Reticulocyte count | Morphology | Etiology | Examples |
| --- | --- | --- | --- |
| Decreased | Hypochromic, microcytic | 1. Impaired Hgb synthesis<br>2. Protoporphyrin deficiency<br>3. Globin synthesis deficiency | 1. Fe deficiency<br>2. Sideroblastic anemia<br>3. Thalassemias |

#### *10.1.2.2. Nuclear maturation defect*

| Reticulocyte count | Morphology | Etiology | Examples |
| --- | --- | --- | --- |
| Decreased | Megaloblastic | DNA synthesis defects | $B_{12}$, folate deficiencies |

## 10.1.3. Survival defect

### 10.1.3.1. Intrinsic (inherited)

| Reticulocyte count | Morphology | Etiology | Examples |
|---|---|---|---|
| Increased | Specific changes | 1. Membrane cytoskeleton protein | 1. Spherocytosis, elliptocytosis |
| | | 2. Metabolic enzymes | 2. $G_6PD$ deficiency |
| | | 3. Hemoglobinopathies | 3. SS disease, HbC, D, E |

### 10.1.3.2. Extrinsic (acquired)

| Reticulocyte count | Morphology | Etiology | Examples |
|---|---|---|---|
| Increased | Specific changes | | Autoimmune hemolysis, malaria, DIC and vascular hemolysis |

## 10.2. The Peripheral Smear—Significance of Specific Changes

### 10.2.1. RBC fragments (schistocytes)

Seen in:
- Microangiopathic hemolytic anemia (TTP, HUS, HEELP and DIC)
- Severe burns
- Valve hemolysis.

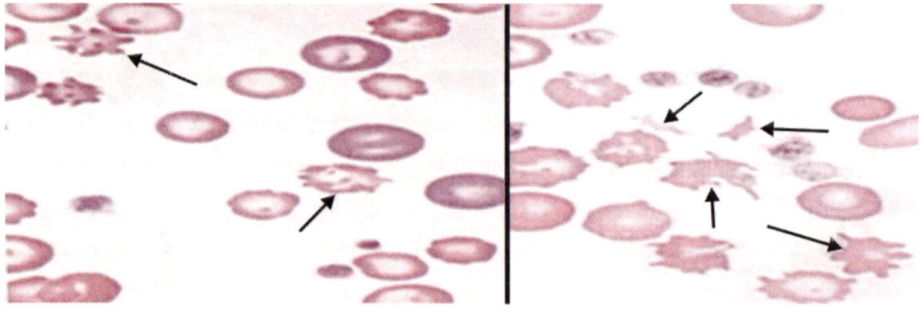

**Fig. 10.1**: Schistocytes

## 10.2.2. Spherocytosis

Seen in:
- Autoimmune hemolytic anemia
- Hereditary spherocytosis.

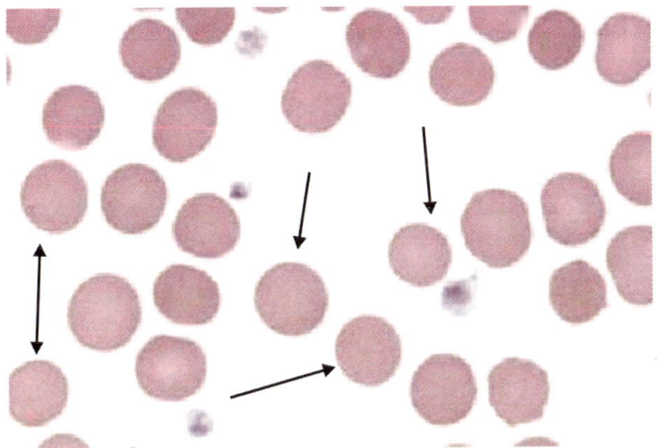

**Fig. 10.2**: Spherocyte

## 10.2.3. Target cells

Seen in:
- Alcoholic or other significant liver disease
- Thalassemia and other hemoglobinopathies (HbC).

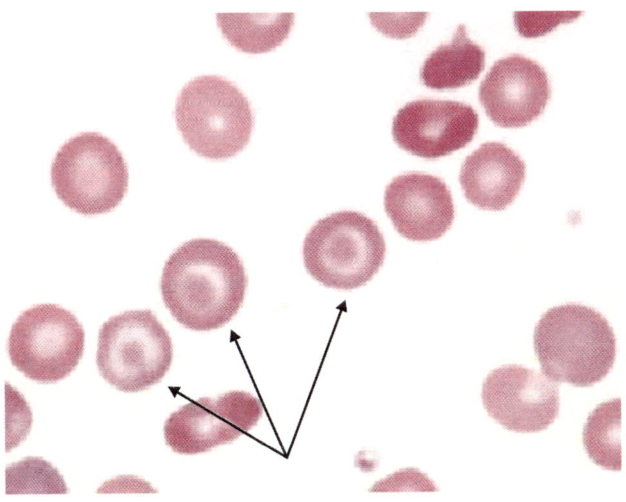

**Fig. 10.3**: Target cell

### 10.2.4. Sideroblasts

Seen in:
- Alcoholic
- Myelodysplasia

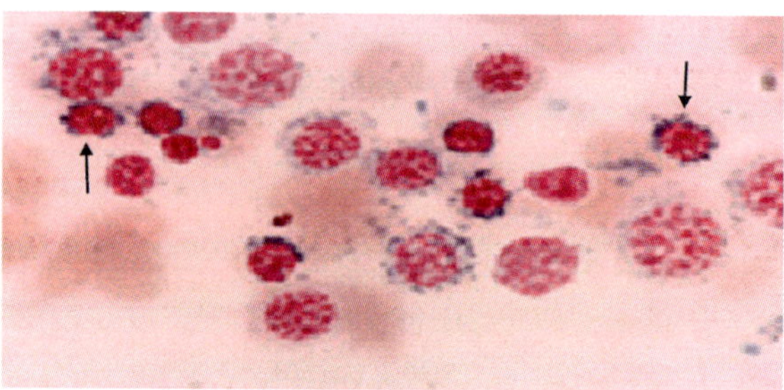

**Fig. 10.4**: Sideroblast

### 10.2.5. Teardrop cells

Seen in:
- Myelofibrosis/myeloid metaplasia
- Thalassemia.

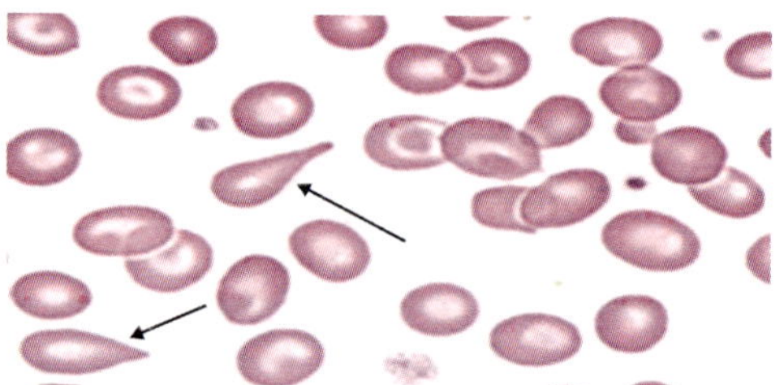

**Fig. 10.5**: Teardrop cell

### 10.2.6. Burr cells (echinocytes)

Seen in:
- Uremic patient.

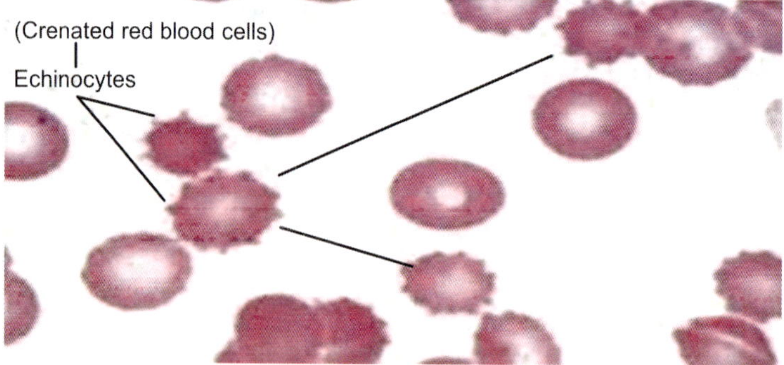


**Fig. 10.6**: Burr cell (echinocyte)

### 10.2.7. Spur cells (acanthocytes)

Seen in:
- Liver disease.

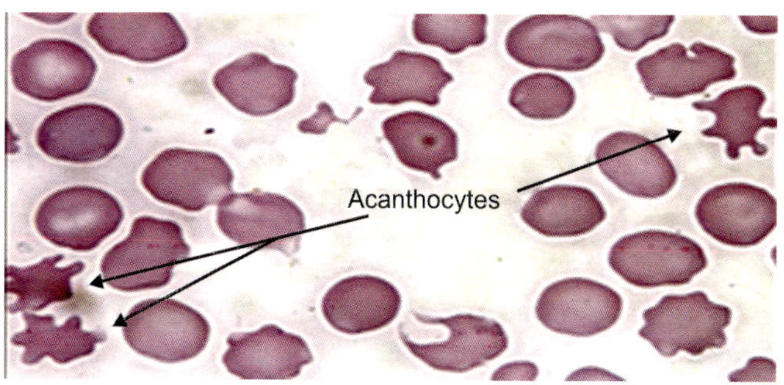



**Fig. 10.7**: Spur cell (acanthocyte)

### 10.2.8. Howell-Jolly bodies

Seen in:
- Splenectomy
- Functional asplenia.

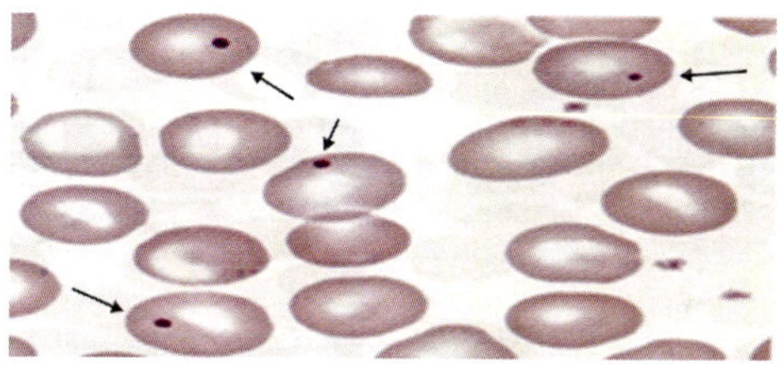

**Fig. 10.8**: Howell-Jolly body

### 10.2.9. Hypersigmented PMNs

Seen in:
Megaloblastic anemia:
- Pernicious anemia
- $B_{12}$ deficiency
- Folate deficiency.

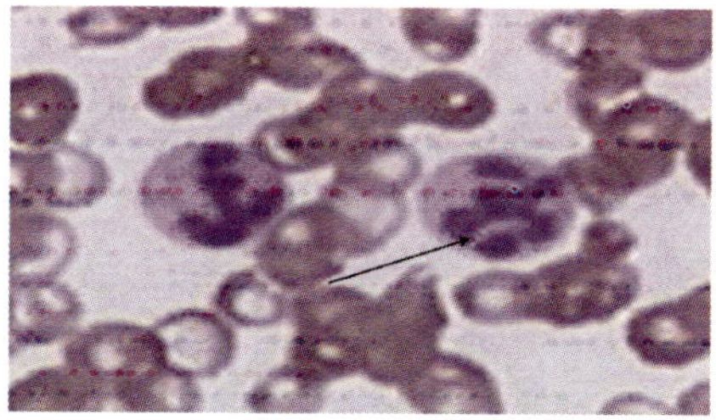

**Fig. 10.9**: Hypersigmented PMNs

## 10.2.10. Some other RBCs shapes

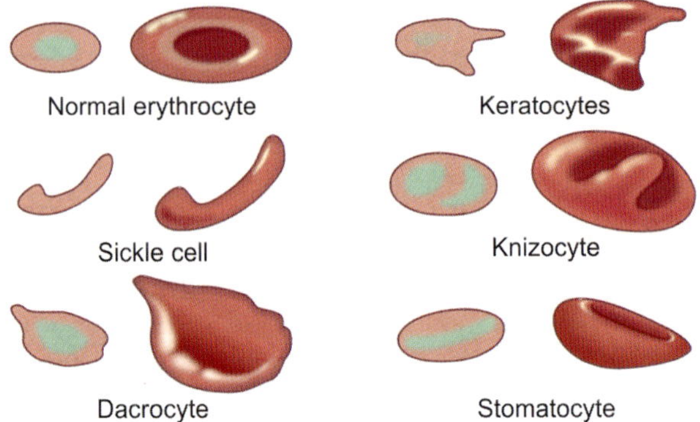


**Fig. 10.10**: Various RBCs shapes

## 10.3. Anemia due to Iron Deficiency vs. Anemia of Chronic Inflammatory Disease (ACD)

|  | Fe deficiency | ACD |
|---|---|---|
| Fe | Low | Low |
| TIBC | High | Low |
| Transferrin saturation | Low | Low to normal |
| Ferritin | Low | Normal to high |

## 10.4. Lab Results of Bleeding Disorders

| | | |
|---|---|---|
| 1. | Elevated PT and PTT | Factor deficiency from common pathway; multiple factor deficiency |
| 2. | Elevated PT normal PTT | Factor VII deficiency |
| 3. | Elevated PTT normal PT—Corrected by addition of plasma | Factor VIII, IX, or XII deficiency |
| 4. | Elevated PTT normal PT—Not corrected by addition of plasma | Inhibitor syndrome (circulating anticoagulant) |
| 5. | Elevated PTT normal PT—But no clinical bleeding disorder | Factor XII deficiency |
| 6. | Normal except elevated bleeding time | Platelet problem |
| i. | Elevated bleeding time with normal platelet aggregation | von Willebrand disease |
| ii. | Elevated bleeding time with abnormal platelet aggregation and decreased platelet count | Bernard-Soulier (giant platelet) syndrome |
| iii. | Elevated bleeding time with abnormal platelet aggregation | Glanzmann thrombasthenia |

## 10.5. Lab Results in DIC

- PT and PTT prolonged
- Thrombocytopenia
- Fibrinogen decreased
- D-dimer increased
- Increased thrombin time
- RBC fragments (schistocytes).

## 10.6.  Use of the Mean Corpuscular Volume (MCV) and Reticulocyte Count in the Diagnosis of Anemia

| Microcytic | |
|---|---|
| **Reticulocyte count** | |
| ↓ | ↓ |
| **Low/inadequate** | **High** |
| • Iron deficiency | • Thalassemia syndrome |
| • Thalassemia trait | • Hemoglobin C and E disorders |
| • Chronic disease/inflammation | • Pyropoikilocytosis |
| • Lead poisoning | |
| • Sideroblastic anemia | |
| • Copper deficiency | |

| Normocytic | |
|---|---|
| **Reticulocyte count** | |
| ↓ | ↓ |
| **Low/inadequate** | **High** |
| • Chronic disease/inflammation | • Antibody-mediated hemolysis |
| • RBC aplasia (TEC, infection, drugs) | • Hypersplenism |
| • Malignancy | • Microagiopathy (HUS, TTP and DIC) |
| • Endocrinopathies | • Membranopathies (spherocytosis, elliptocytosis and ovalocytosis) |
| • Renal failure | • Enzymopathies (G6PD and PK deficiencies) |
| • Acute bleeding | • Hemangiopathies (HbSS and SC) |
| • Hypersplenism | |
| • Dyserythropoietic anemia II | |
| • Hemophagocytic syndrome | |

| Macrocytic | |
|---|---|
| **Reticulocyte count** | |
| ↓ | ↓ |
| **Low/inadequate** | **High** |
| – Folate deficiency<br>– Vitamin $B_{12}$ deficiency<br><br>– Acquired aplastic anemia<br>– Congenital aplastic anemia (Diamond-Blackfan, Fanconi anemia, Pearson syndrome)<br>– Drug-induced<br>– Trisomy 21<br>– Hypothyroidism<br>– Orotic aciduria | – Dyserythropoietic anemia I and III<br>– Active hemolysis with very high reticulocyte count |

## 10.7. Hematology and Laboratory Features of Congenital Dyserythropoietic Anemia

| Test | CDA 1 | CDA 2 | CDA 3 |
|---|---|---|---|
| Blood smear | Anisopoikilocytosis Basophilic stippling Occasional circulating mature erythroblast | Anisopoikilocytosis Basophilic stippling Occasional circulating mature erythroblast | Anisopoikilo-cytosis Basophilic stippling |
| Hgb (g/dL) | 6.5–11.5 (mean = 9.5) | 9–12 (mean = 11) | 8–14 (mean = 12) |
| MCV | ↑↑ (70% cases) | Normal or minimum ↑ | Normal or minimum ↑ |
| RDW | ↑↑↑ | ↑↑ | ↑↑ |
| Reticulocyte | Suboptimal response | – | N/A |
| Bilirubin (total, mg/dL) | ↑ (indirect) | ↑ (2–8) | Normal or minimum ↑ |
| LDH | ↑ | ↑ | ↑↑↑ |
| Haptoglobin | N/A | – | ↓ or absent |
| Ferritin (µg/L) | ↑ (in 60% = 1000–1500) | ↑↑ (>50% >1000 by age 50 years) | N |
| Ham (acid sera-lysis) test | Negative | Positive | Negative |
| Anti-i antigen hemagglutination | Normal to strong | Strong | Normal to strong |
| Serum thymidine kinase | ↑↑↑ | ↑↑ | ↑↑↑ |
| SDS-PAGE | Normal | Abnormal migration of band-3 | Normal |
| Hemosiderinuria | N/A | N/A | +++ |

## 10.8. Laboratory Studies Differentiating the Most Common Microcytic Anemias

| Study | Iron deficiency anemia | α or β thalassemia | Anemia of chronic disease |
|---|---|---|---|
| Hemoglobin | Decreased | Decreased | Decreased |
| RDW | Increased | Normal | Normal-increased |
| RBC | Decreased | Normal-increased | Normal-decreased |
| Serum ferritin | Decreased | Normal | Increased |
| Total Fe binding capacity | Increased | Normal | Decreased |
| Transferrin saturation | Decreased | Normal | Decreased |
| FEP | Increased | Normal | Increased |
| Transferrin receptor | Increased | Normal | Increased |
| Reticulocyte hemoglobin concentration | Decreased | Normal | Normal-decreased |

## 10.9. Selected Cutoff Values to Define Iron Deficiency Anemia

| Indicator | Selected cutoff values to define iron deficiency |
|---|---|
| Hemoglobin (g/L) | 6 month–5 year <110, 6–11 year <115 |
| Mean corpuscular volume (MCV) ($\mu m^3$) | Children older than 11 year and adults <82 |
| Reticulocyte hemoglobin content (CHr) (pg.) | In infants and young children <27.5 |
| Erythrocyte zinc protoporphyrin (ZPP) ($\mu mol/mol$ heme) | ≤5 year >70, children >5 year >80 children >5 year on washed red cells >40 |
| Transferrin saturation | <16% |
| Serum ferritin (SF) ($\mu g/L$) | ≤5 year <12, children >5 year <15 In all age groups in the presence of infection <30 |
| Serum transferrin receptor (sTfR) | Cutoff varies with assay and with patient's age and ethnic origin |

## 10.10. Possible Complications of Blood Transfusions

| The complications can be broadly classified into two categories: | |
| --- | --- |
| **A.  Immune complications** | |
| **1.  Hemolytic complications**<br><br>    a.  **Acute hemolytic reactions:**<br><br>        i.  Usually due to ABO blood type incompatibility<br><br>        ii.  Human error plays a large part in these reactions | **2.  Nonhemolytic complications**<br><br>    i.  Due to sensitization of the recipient to donor white cells, platelets or plasma proteins |
| b.  Delayed hemolytic reactions:<br><br>        i.  Generally mild in comparison<br><br>        ii.  Caused by antibodies to non-D antigens of the Rh system or to foreign alleles in other systems such as the Kell, Duffy or Kidd antigens | ii.  These reactions include:<br>• Febrile<br>• Urticarial<br>• Anaphylactic<br>• Pulmonary edema (non-cardiogenic)<br>• Graft vs host<br>• Purpura<br>• Immune suppression |
| **B.  Nonimmune complications** | |
| The nonimmune complications can also be classified into two broad categories: | |
| a.  **Complications associated with massive blood transfusion**<br><br>• Coagulopathy<br>• Citrate toxicity<br>• Hypothermia<br>• Acid-base disturbances<br>• Changes in serum potassium concentration | b.  **Infectious complications**<br><br>• Hepatitis<br>• AIDS<br>• Other viral agents (CMV, EBV, HTLV)<br>• Parasites and bacteria |

## 10.11. Inherited Causes of Lymphocytopenia

- Aplasia of lymphopoietic stem cells
- Severe combined immunodeficiency
- Ataxia-telangiectasia
- Wiskott-Aldrich syndrome
- Immunodeficiency with thymoma
- Cartilage-hair hypoplasia
- Idiopathic CD4 T lymphocytopenia.

## 10.12. Causes of Red Cell Fragmentation Syndromes

Microangiopathic:
    i. Hemolytic uremic syndrome
    ii. Thrombotic thrombocytopenic purpura
    iii. Meningococcal sepsis
    iv. Disseminated intravascular coagulation.
Cardiac valves or arterial grafts
March hemoglobinuria
Infections—Malaria and clostridia
Chemical and physical burns
Liver and renal disease.

## 10.13. Causes of a Raised Platelet Count (Thrombocytosis)

In children nearly always reactive or secondary:
    i. Infection
    ii. Iron deficiency
    iii. Postoperative
    iv. Inflammation
    v. Malignancy
    vi. Hemorrhage.
Primary disease of the marrow is very rare.

## 10.14. Causes of Thrombocytopenia

Decreased production:
    Congenital—Rare
    Acquired.
Increased destruction:
    Immune (common).
    Nonimmune:
        Disseminated intravascular coagulation
        Hemolytic uremic syndrome and its variants
        Hypersplenism.

## 10.15. Causes of Immune Thrombocytopenia

Idiopathic autoimmune (ITP or AITP):
    Acute (80–90% in children)
    Chronic (i.e. > 6 months' duration).
Alloantibodies:
    Neonatal (NAIT)
    Post-transfusion purpura

Drug-induced.

Disease-associated:

For example

   i.  Systemic lupus erythematosus

  ii.  Immunodeficiency

 iii.  Some infections.

### 10.16.  Hemophilia A and B—Level of Clotting Factor Related to Clinical Features

| Level of clotting factor (% of normal) | Clinical features |
|---|---|
| <1% | Severe disease<br>Spontaneous bleeding into joints and muscles |
| 1–5% | Moderate disease<br>Bleeding after trauma<br>Occasional spontaneous bleeding |
| 5–40% | Mild disease<br>Bleeding after trauma |

### 10.17. Complications Associated with Sickle Cell Trait

| | |
|---|---|
| Renal medullary cancer | Splenic infarction |
| Hematuria | Exertional rhabdomyolysis |
| Renal papillary necrosis | Exercise-related sudden death |
| Hyposthenuria | Protection against severe falciparum malaria |

### Bibliography


1. http://emedicine.medscape.com/article/202333-overview
2. http://my.clevelandclinic.org/disorders/immune_thrombocytopenic_purpura_itp
3. http://www.cdc.gov/ncbddd/hemophilia/facts.html
4. http://www.haematologica.org/content/95/6/1034.full
5. http://www.idph.state.il.us/HealthWellness/sicklecell.htm
6. http://www.ihaematology.com/general-haematology/laboratory-haematology
7. http://www.wheelessonline.com/ortho/12795

# Infectious Diseases

## 11.1. Diagnostic Criteria of Staphylococcal Toxic Shock Syndrome

Major criteria (all required)
i. Acute fever; temperature >38.8°C.
ii. Hypotension (orthostatic and shock; below age—Appropriate norms).
iii. Rash (erythroderma with convalescent desquamation).

Minor criteria (any 3 or more)
i. Mucous membrane inflammation (vaginal, oropharyngeal or conjunctival hyperemia, and strawberry tongue).
ii. Vomiting and diarrhea.
iii. Liver abnormalities (bilirubin or transaminase greater than twice upper limit of normal).
iv. Renal abnormalities (urea nitrogen or creatinine greater than twice upper limit of normal, or greater than 5 white blood cells per high power field).
v. Muscle abnormalities (myalgia or creatinine phosphokinase greater than twice upper limit of normal).
vi. Central nervous system abnormalities (alteration in consciousness without focal neurological signs).
vii. Thrombocytopenia ($100,000/mm^3$ or less).

Exclusionary criteria
i. Absence of another explanation.
ii. Negative blood cultures (except occasionally for *Staphylococcus aureus*).

## 11.2. Diphtheria

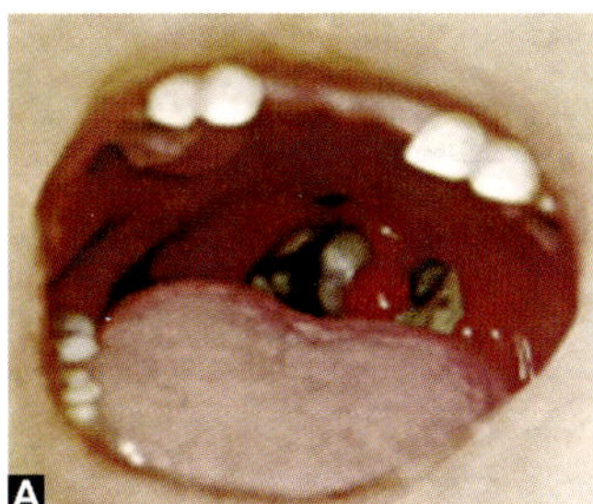 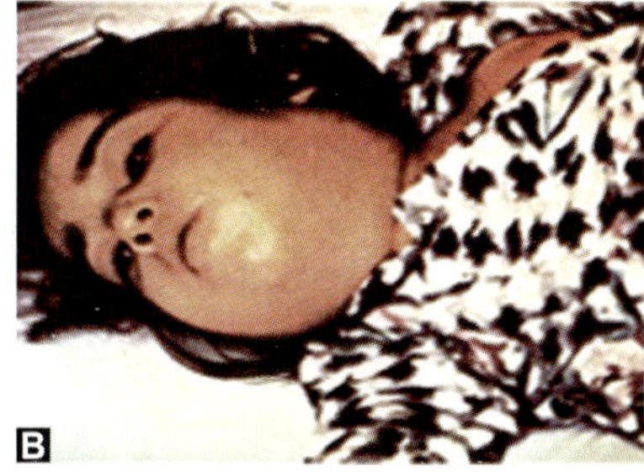

**Figs 11.1A and B**: Diphtheria. A: Tonsillar diphtheria and B: Bull-neck appearance of diphtheritic cervical lymphadenopathy

## 11.3. Late Manifestations of Congenital Syphilis

| Symptoms/signs | Description |
| --- | --- |
| Olympian brow | Bony prominence of the forehead due to persistent or recurrent periostitis |
| Clavicular or Higouménaki sign | Unilateral or bilateral thickening of the sternoclavicular third of the clavicle |
| Saber shins | Anterior bowing of the midportion of the tibia |
| Scaphoid scapula | Convexity along the medial border of the scapula |
| Hutchinson teeth | Peg-shaped upper central incisors; they erupt during 6 years of life with abnormal enamel, resulting in a notch along the biting surface |
| Mulberry molars | Abnormal 1st lower (6 years) molars characterized by small biting surface and excessive number of cusps |
| Saddle nose | Depression of the nasal root, a result of syphilitic rhinitis destroying adjacent bone and cartilage |
| Rhagades | Linear scars that extend in a spoke-like pattern from previous mucocutaneous fissures of the mouth, anus and genitalia |
| Juvenile paresis | Latent meningovascular infection; it is rare and typically occurs during adolescence with behavioral changes, focal seizures, or loss of intellectual function |
| Juvenile tabes | Rare spinal cord involvement and cardiovascular involvement with aortitis |
| Hutchinson triad | Hutchinson teeth, interstitial keratitis, and eighth nerve deafness |
| Clutton joint | Unilateral or bilateral painless joint swelling (usually involving knees) due to synovitis with sterile synovial fluid; spontaneous remission usually occurs after several week |
| Interstitial keratitis | Manifests with intense photophobia and lacrimation, followed within weeks or months by corneal opacification and complete blindness |
| Eighth nerve deafness | May be unilateral or bilateral, appears at any age, manifests initially as vertigo and high-tone hearing loss, and progresses to permanent deafness |

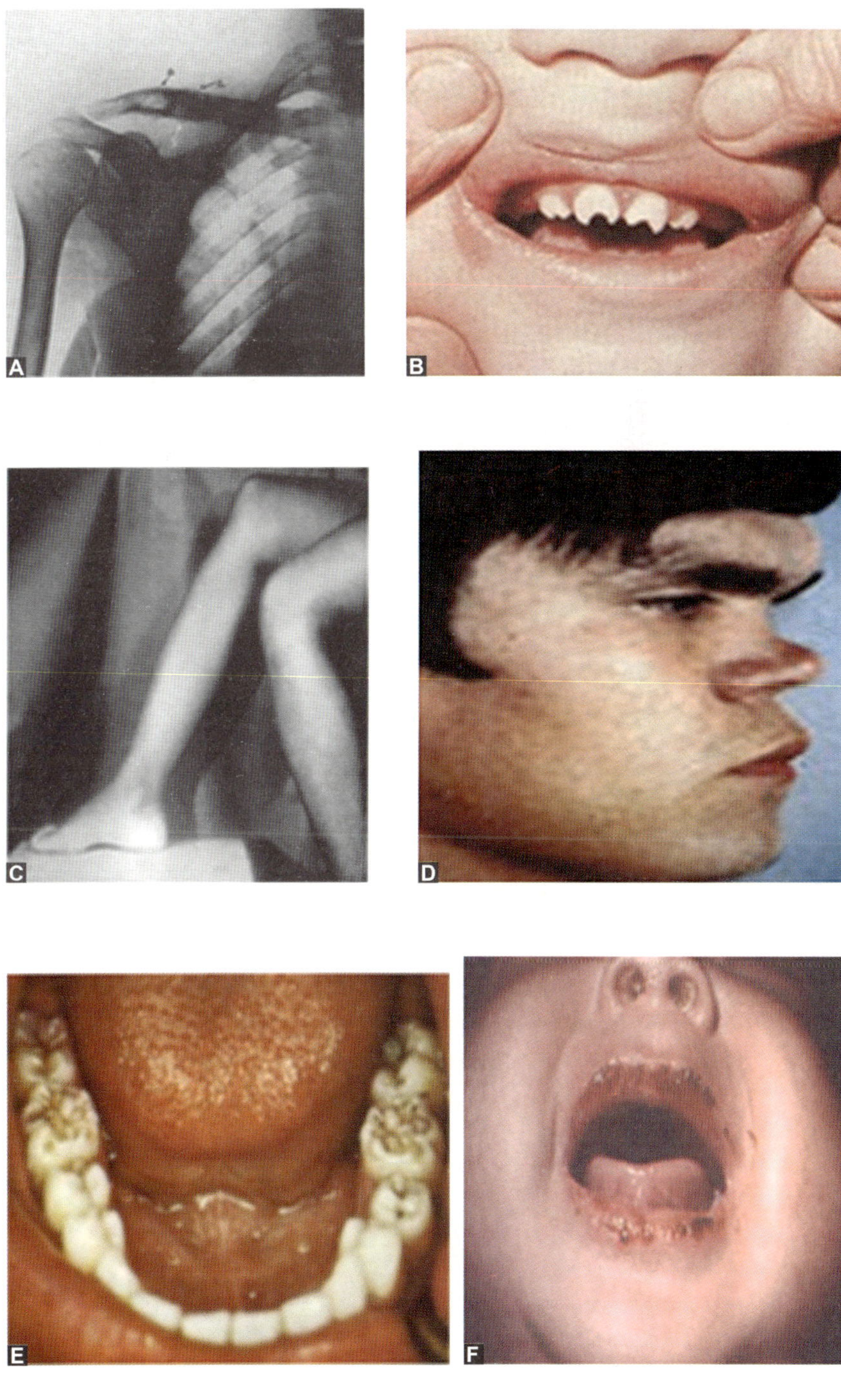

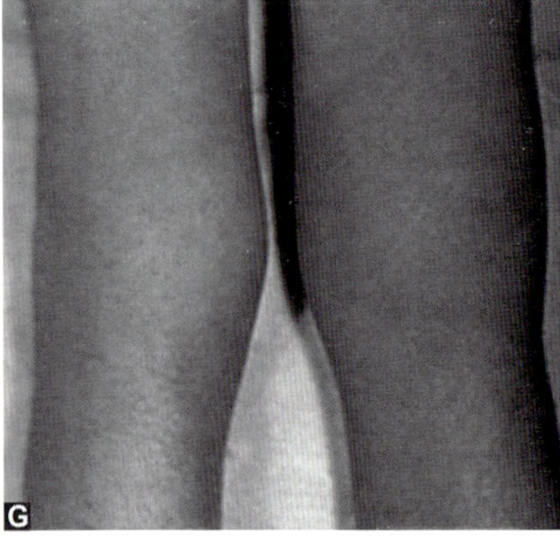 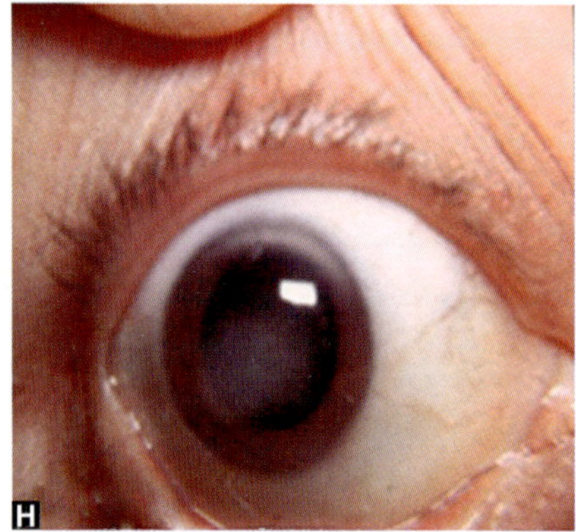

**Figs 11.2A to H**: Various signs of congenital syphilis: (A) Clavicular or Higouménakis sign, (B) Hutchinson teeth, (C) Saber shins, (D) Saddle nose, (E) Mulberry molars, (F) Rhagades, (G) Clutton joint and (H) Interstitial keratitis

## 11.4. Definition of Streptococcal Toxic Shock Syndrome

### Clinical criteria

- Hypotension plus 2 or more of the following:
  - Renal impairment
  - Coagulopathy
  - Hepatic impairment
  - Generalized erythematous macular rash
  - Soft tissue necrosis.

### Definite case

- Clinical criteria plus group A streptococcus from a normally sterile site.

### Probable case

- Clinical criteria plus group A streptococcus from a nonsterile site.

## 11.5. Children At High-risk of Invasive Pneumococcal Infection

- **Children with:**
  - Sickle cell disease congenital or acquired asplenia or splenic dysfunction.
  - Human immunodeficiency virus infection.
  - Cochlear implants.

## 11.6. Scarlet Fever

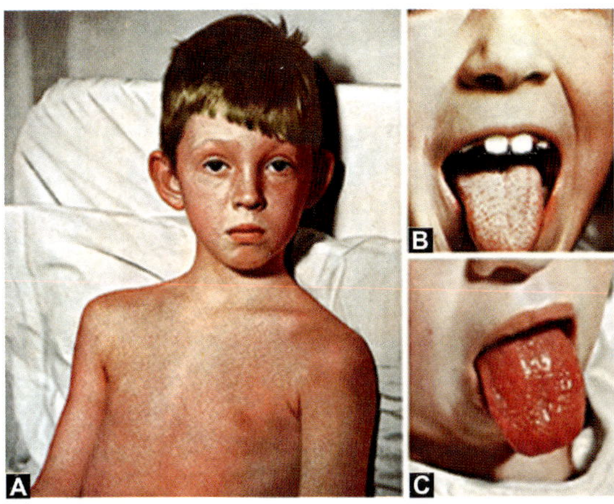

**Figs 11.3A to C**: Scarlet fever: A: Punctate, erythematous rash (2nd day), B: White strawberry tongue (1st day) and C: Red strawberry tongue (3rd day)

### Scarlet fever

- It is an upper respiratory tract infection associated with a characteristic rash, which is caused by an infection with pyrogenic exotoxin (erythrogenic toxin)-producing Group A streptococcus (GAS) in individuals who do not have antitoxin antibodies.
- The milder form with equivocal pharyngeal findings can be confused with:
  - i. Viral exanthems
  - ii. Kawasaki disease
  - iii. Drug eruptions.

## 11.7. Pathophysiologic Events in Postnatally Acquired Rubella Virus Infection

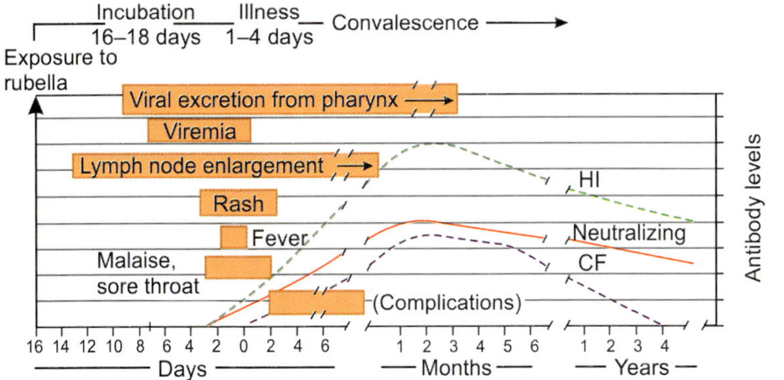


**Fig. 11.4**: Rubella; graph of pathophysiologic events

### 11.7.1. Complications of postnatally acquired rubella virus infection

Possible complications include:
1.  Arthralgia and/or arthritis
2.  Thrombocytopenic purpura
3.  Encephalitis.

## 11.8.    Schematic Representation of the Development of Antibodies to Various Epstein-Barr Virus Antigens in Patients with Infectious Mononucleosis

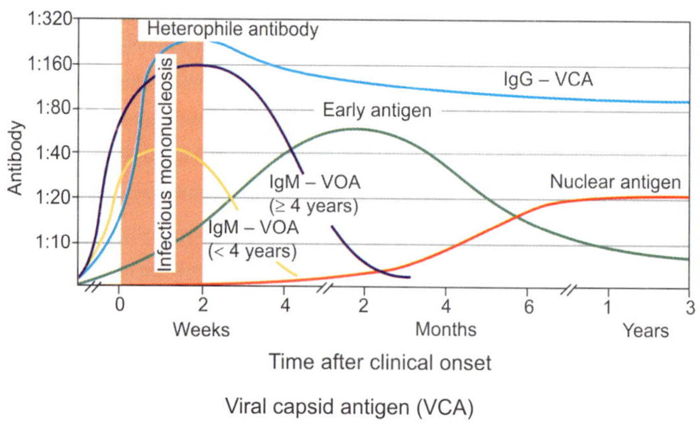


**Fig. 11.5**: Infectious mononucleosis; Epstein-Barr virus antigens

## 11.9.    Pathophysiologic Events in Measles, Rubella, Scarlet Fever and Roseola Infantum

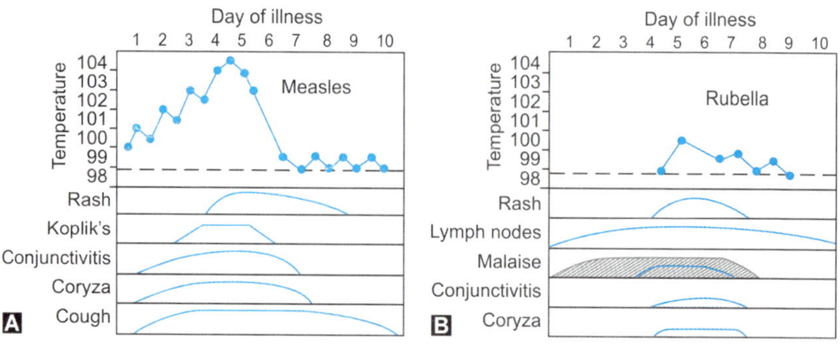

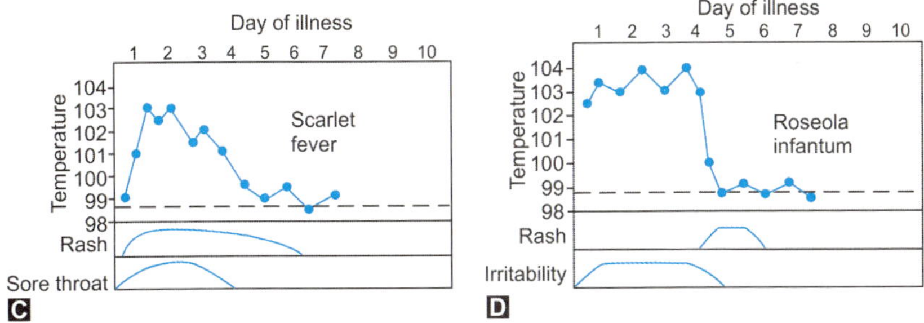

**Figs 11.6A to D**: Pathophysiologic events in A: measles, B: rubella,
C: scarlet fever and D: roseola infantum

## 11.10. Complications of Infectious Mononucleosis

1. Respiratory complications:
   Airway obstruction (drooling, stridor, and interference with breathing).
2. Subcapsular splenic hemorrhage or splenic rupture
   (Most feared complication) (2nd week of illness).
3. Neurological complications:
   i. Severe neurologic manifestations, such as seizures and ataxia, in 1–5% of cases.
   ii. Alice in Wonderland syndrome (metamorphopsia) perceptual distortions of sizes, shapes, and spatial relationships.
   iii. Meningitis with nuchal rigidity and mononuclear cells in the cerebrospinal fluid.
   iv. Facial nerve palsy.
   v. Transverse myelitis.
   vi. Encephalitis.
4. Guillain-Barré syndrome or Reye syndrome may follow acute illness.
5. Hematological complications:
   i. Hemolytic anemia, often with a positive Coombs test result and with cold agglutinins specific for RBC i antigen
      – Occurs in 3% of cases
      – The onset is typically in the first 2 weeks of illness and lasts <1 month.
   ii. Mild thrombocytopenia and neutropenia are common, severe thrombocytopenia (<20,000 platelets/dL) or severe neutropenia (<1,000 neutrophils/dL) is rare.
   iii. Aplastic anemia is a rare complication that usually manifests 3–4 weeks after the onset of illness, usually with recovery in 4–8 days, but some cases do require bone marrow transplantation.
6. Myocarditis or interstitial pneumonia may occur, and both resolve in 3–4 weeks.
7. Other rare complications are pancreatitis, parotitis and orchitis.

## 11.11. Definition of Positive Tuberculin Skin Testing

**Induration ≥ 5 mm**

- Children in close contact with known or suspected contagious cases of tuberculosis.
- Children suspected to have tuberculosis based on clinical or radiographic findings.
- Children on immunosuppressive therapy or with immunosuppressive conditions (including HIV infection).

**Induration ≥ 10 mm**

- Children at increased risk for dissemination based on young age (<4 years) or with other medical conditions (cancer, diabetes mellitus, chronic renal failure, or malnutrition).
- Children with increased exposure: Those born in or whose parents were born in endemic countries; those with travel to endemic countries; those exposed to HIV-infected adults, homeless persons, illicit drug users.

**Induration ≥ 15 mm**

- Children ≥ 4 years without any risk factors.

## 11.12. Clinical Features of Congenital Rubella, Cytomegalovirus and Toxoplasmosis

|  | Cytomegalovirus | Rubella | Toxoplasmosis |
|---|---|---|---|
| CNS |  |  |  |
| Hydrocephaly | + | – | +++ |
| Microcephaly | + | +++ | – |
| Calcification | +++ | + | ++ |
| Deafness | ++ | +++ | ++ |
| Encephalitis | – | – | + |
| Eyes |  |  |  |
| Microphthalmia | + | + | +++ |
| Cataracts | – | ++ | + |
| Chorioretinitis | + | + | +++ |
| Intrauterine growth retardation | + | +++ | + |
| Cardiac lesion | – | ++ | + |
| Purpuric rash | ++ | +++ | – |
| Pneumonia | +++ | ++ | ++ |
| Hepatosplenomegaly | ++ | +++ | ++++ |
| Lymphadenopathy | – | – | + |
| Bony lesion | + | +++ | – |

## 11.13. Mechanisms of Bacterial Resistance to Antibiotics

Bacteria acquire resistance to antibiotics most commonly by one of three main mechanisms—

1. Inability to reach the site of action due to decreased cell wall permeability or increased action of efflux pumps.
   Examples of this type of mechanism occur in Pseudomonas spp. and Enterobacteriaceae as a mechanism of resistance to aminoglycosides.
2. Alteration in the antimicrobial target.
   An example is alteration in the penicillin-binding protein 2 in staphylococci to PBP-2a encoded by the mec A gene, which renders all $\beta$-lactam antibiotics, including the penicillinase-resistant penicillins, inactive, i.e. MRSA.
3. Production of an enzyme that inactivates the antibiotic.
   Examples are $\beta$-lactamases, which cleave the $\beta$-lactam ring and render these antibiotics inactive.

## 11.14. Recommendation of Usage of Pneumococcal Polysaccharide Vaccines (PPV)

PPV is recommended as an additional strategy for children aged 2 years or older in whom pneumococcal infection is likely to be more common and/or dangerous

- Asplenia or severe dysfunction of the spleen, e.g. homozygous sickle cell disease and celiac syndrome.
- Chronic renal disease or nephrotic syndrome.
- Immunodeficiency or immunosuppression from disease or treatment (including HIV infection).
- Chronic heart, lung or liver disease.
- Diabetes mellitus.
- Cochlear implants.
- History of invasive pneumococcal disease.
- Presence of CSF shunt or other condition with risk of CSF leak.

## 11.15. Factors Associated with Mother-to-Child Transmission (MTCT) of HIV

- Without interventions, the rate of MTCT was 15–20% in Europe and 25 – 40% in Africa.
- Most MTCT occurs around the time of delivery.
- Increased risk is associated with:
  - Late stage maternal disease
  - High maternal plasma viremia
  - Prolonged rupture of membranes

– Invasive obstetric procedures
– Prematurity
– Breastfeeding.

## Bibliography

1. http://www.cdc.gov/tb/publications/factsheets/testing/skintesting.htm
2. http://www.cdc.gov/vaccines/vpd-vac/diphtheria
3. http://www.hopkinsmedicine.org/healthlibrary/conditions/infectious_ diseases/infectious_mononucleosis_
4. http://www.moleculartb.org/gb/pdf/transcriptions/11_YZhang.pdf
5. http://www.nc.cdc.gov/eid/article/1/3/pdfs/95-0301.pdf
6. http://www.who.int/ith/diseases/pneumococcal/en/index.html
7. http://www.who.int/reproductivehealth/topics/rtis/syphilis/en/

# Metabolic Disorders

## 12.1. Suspicion of Inborn Errors

Suspicion of inborn errors if encephalopathy occurs in neonates or young infants or occurs suddenly without warning and progress rapidly.

Because of acute onset, it is usually not associated with focal neurologic deficits.

### 12.1.1. Symptoms can include

- Unexplained seizures
- Coma
- Lethargy
- Hypertonia
- Hypotonia.

### 12.1.2. Examples of the most common, associated diseases are

- Maple syrup urine disease
- Ornithine  transcarbamoylase (OTC) deficiency
- Propionic acidemia.

Most of these infants are normal at birth.

## 12.2.  The Classical Galactosemia (Deficiency of Galactose-1-Phosphate Uridyltransferase)

The infant cannot metabolize galactose -1-phosphate, and this accumu-lates in the kidney, liver and brain.

### 12.2.1. The signs and symptoms of classic galactosemia include

#### 12.2.1.1  Galactosemia include:

| | |
|---|---|
| Jaundice | Vomiting |
| Hepatosplenomegaly | Seizures |
| Hypoglycemia | Lethargy |
| Irritability | Poor weight gain |
| Cataracts | Vitreous hemorrhage |
| Cirrhosis | Ascites |
| Mental retardation | Vomiting |

## 12.3. Friedreich Ataxia

### 12.3.1. Facts about Friedreich ataxia

- AR
- Mapped on chromosome 9
- Occurs in about 1/50,000.

### 12.3.2. Symptoms include

- Hypoactive or absent deep tendon reflexes
- Ataxia
- Corticospinal tract dysfunction
- Impaired vibratory and proprioceptive function
- Hypertrophic cardiomyopathy
- Diabetes mellitus.

## 12.4. Recognition Pattern of Mucopolysaccharidosis

| Manifestations | Mucopolysaccharidosis type | | | | | | |
|---|---|---|---|---|---|---|---|
| | I-H | I-S | II | III | IV | VI | VII |
| Mental deficiency | + | − | ± | + | − | − | ± |
| Coarse facial features | + | (+) | + | + | − | + | ± |
| Corneal clouding | + | + | − | − | (+) | + | + |
| Visceromegaly | + | (+) | + | (+) | − | + | + |
| Short stature | + | (+) | + | − | + | + | + |
| Joint contractures | + | + | + | − | − | + | + |
| Dysostosis multiplex | + | (+) | + | (+) | + | + | + |
| Leukocyte inclusions | + | (+) | + | + | − | + | + |
| Mucopolysacchariduria | + | + | + | + | + | + | + |

I-H—Hurler disease; I-S—Scheie disease; II—Hunter disease; III—Sanfilippo disease; IV—Morquio disease; VI—Maroteaux-Lamy; VII—Sly disease

## 12.5. Mucopolysaccharidosis Type I (Hurler Syndrome)

### 12.5.1. Facts about Hurler syndrome

- MPS I is caused by mutations of the IUA gene on chromosome 4p16.3 encoding $\alpha$-L-iduronidase.
- An infant with Hurler syndrome appears normal at birth, but inguinal hernias are often present.
- Is a severe, progressive disorder with multiple organ and tissue involvement that results in premature death, usually by 10 year of age.
- Diagnosis is usually made between 6 and 24 months of age.

## 12.5.2. Common findings in Hurler syndrome

| | |
|---|---|
| Hepatosplenomegaly | Prominent forehead |
| Coarse facial features | Joint stiffness |
| Corneal clouding | Short stature |
| Large tongue | Skeletal dysplasia |

## 12.6. Mucopolysaccharidosis Type II (Hunter Syndrome)

### 12.6.1. Facts about Hunter syndrome

- Due to defect in the gene that encodes for iduronate-2-sulfatase on chromosome Xq27–28.
- Only males are affected.
- In severely affected children, diagnosis is usually made by 2 years of age.

### 12.6.2. Common findings in Hunter syndrome

| | |
|---|---|
| Learning difficulties (with challenging behavior, ADD, or seizures) | Nodular rash around the scapulae and the extensor surfaces is pathognomonic (rare in children) |
| Middle ear diseases | Joint stiffness |
| Hernias | Hepatosplenomegaly |
| Coarse facial appearance | Diarrhea |

## 12.7. Phenylketonuria (PKU)

- AR disorder
- Phenylalanine cannot be converted to tyrosine
- The enzyme defect is phenylalanine hydroxylase (PAH).

The most common presentations in infant include:
- Vomiting.
- Irritability.
- An eczematoid rash.
- Peculiar odor-"mousy", "wolf-like" or musty in character (due to the phenylacetic acid in urine).
- Nearly all are fair-haired and fair-skinned.

## 12.8. Metabolic Screening

- It is not recommended for asymptomatic children with idiopathic mental retardation.
- Consider metabolic screening if the following symptoms are present with mental retardation:
  - Episodic vomiting or lethargy
  - Poor feeding
  - Poor growth
  - Seizures
  - Unusual odors
  - Loss of developmental skills
  - Sensory abnormality (specially retina)
  - Acquired skin disorders.

## 12.9. Some of the Most Common Reasons for Referral to a Metabolic Clinic

Some of the most common reasons for referral to a metabolic clinic are:
- Disorders detected by expanded newborn screening.
- Suspected or confirmed lactic acidosis.
- Suspected or confirmed metabolic neurological disorders; including nonspecific developmental delay.
- Metabolic bone diseases such as nutritional or hereditary rickets.
- Failure to thrive.
- Hypercholesterolemia.
- Suspected porphyria.
- Visceromegaly.

## 12.10. Disorders of Fatty Acid Metabolism

Disorders of fatty acid metabolism commonly present with one of three phenotypes:
1. Sudden infant death.
2. Hypoketotic hypoglycemia in association with recurrent vomiting and hepatic encephalopathy.
3. Recurrent rhabdomyolysis and myoglobinuria.

## 12.11. Inborn Errors of Metabolism that Cause Elevated Blood Lactate

Inborn errors of metabolism that cause  elevated blood lactate include disorders of:

- Pyruvate metabolism and the Krebs cycle
- Gluconeogenesis
- Fatty acid oxidation
- Mitochondrial function
- Organic acid metabolism
- Biotin metabolism
- Glycogen storage diseases.

## 12.12. Flowchart for Differential Diagnosis of Hyperammonemia

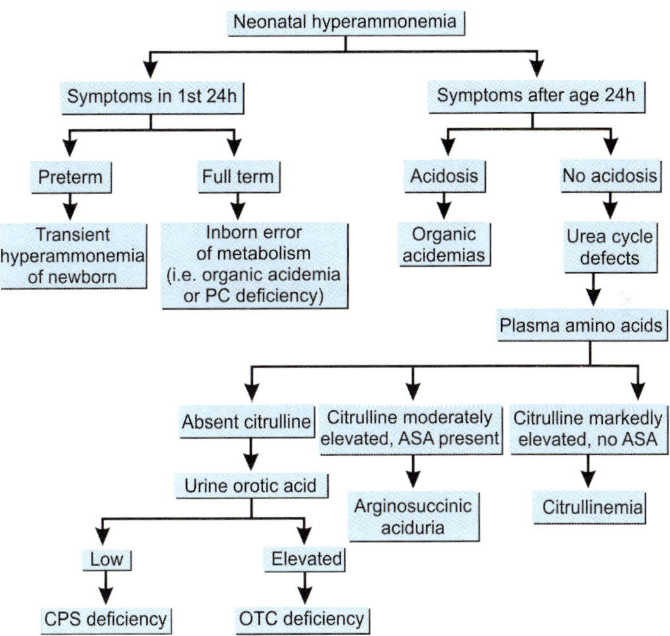


(ASA—Arginosuccinic acid; CPS—Carbamyl phosphate synthetase; OTC—Ornithine transcarbamylase; PC—Pyruvate carboxylase)

### 12.13.  Flowchart for Evaluation of Metabolic Acidosis in the Young Infant

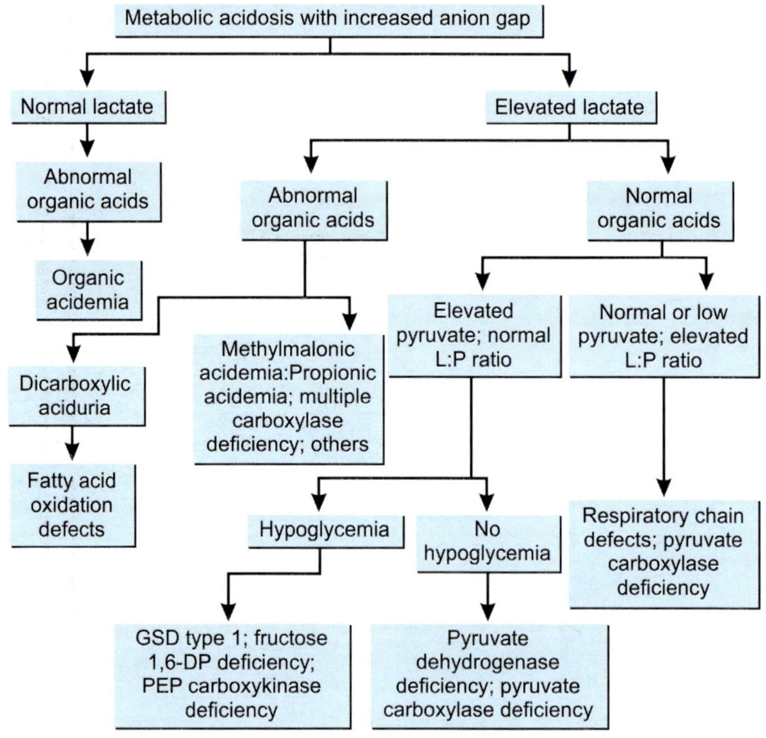



(Fructose-1, 6-DP, fructose-1, 6-diphosphatase; GSD, glycogen storage disease; L : P ratio, lactate to pyruvate ratio

### 12.14.  Special Smell that Indicate the Inborn Error of Metabolisms (IEMs)

| The smell | The inborn error of metabolism |
| --- | --- |
| Musty or Mousy | PKU |
| Boiled cabbage | Tyrosinemia or hypermethioninemia |
| Maple Syrup | Maple syrup urine disease |
| Sweaty feet | Isovaleric acidemia or glutaric acidemia type II |
| Cat urine | Multiple carboxylase deficiencies (biotin deficiency) |

## 12.15. Quick References for Differential Diagnosis of Inborn Error of Metabolism

| Diagnosis / Labtest | Nonketotic hyper-glycemia | Urea-cycle defect | 1. Fatty acid oxidation defects 2. Organic acidemia | Organic acidemia | Organic acidemia | Organic acidemia | 1. Glycogen Storage-defects 2. Amino acidurias 3. Carbohydrate metabolism defect |
|---|---|---|---|---|---|---|---|
| Metabolic acidosis | ↔ | ↔ | ↑ | ↑ | ↑ | ↑ | ↑ |
| Ammonia | ↔ | ↔ | ↑ | ↑ | ↑ | ↔ | ↔ |
| Glucose | ↔ | ↔ | ↓ | ↔ | ↑ | ↔ | ↓ |

## 12.16. Organic Acidemias

*For example*: Methylmalonic or propionic acidemia, multiple carboxylase deficiency.

1. These are caused by abnormal metabolism of proteins, fats or carbohydrates.
2. These are characterized by:
    i. Marked metabolic acidosis with ketosis
    ii. Often with elevated lactate
    iii. Mild to moderate hyperammonemia.
3. Common signs include:
    i. Vomiting
    ii. Signs of encephalopathy
    iii. Neutropenia and thrombocytopenia.

## 12.17. Fatty Acid Oxidation Defects

*For example*: Short, medium and long-chain acyl-CoA dehydrogenase deficiencies (known as β-oxidation defects):

1. These are a distinct type of organic acid disorder, characterized by:
    i. Hypoketotic hypoglycemia
    ii. Hyperammonemia
    iii. Cardiomyopathy.
2. It may present clinically with Reye's syndrome.

3. Medium-chain acyl-CoA dehydrogenase deficiency (MCAD) is among the most common of all IEMs and may account for 5% of SIDS cases.

## 12.18. Primary Lactic Acidosis

*For example*:
  i. Pyruvate dehydrogenase
  ii. Pyruvate carboxylase
  iii. Cytochrome oxidase deficiencies.
   • Present with severe lactic acidosis.

## 12.19. Aminoacidopathies

*For example*:
   i. Phenylketonuria
   ii. Hereditary tyrosinemia
   iii. Nonketotic hyperglycinemia
   iv. Maple syrup urine disease [MSUD]
   v. Homocystinuria .
1. May have similar presentation to the organic acidemias, but are a very heterogeneous group of disorders.
2. Hereditary tyrosinemia can present in the neonate with a bleeding diathesis due to liver disease, or later in infancy with a renal Fanconi syndrome.
3. The severe form of nonketotic hyperglycinemia presents as unremitting seizures with hypotonia and hiccoughs.
4. MSUD classically presents at the end of the first week of life with:
   i. Feeding difficulties
   ii. Lethargy
   iii. Coma
   iv. Seizures
   v. Characteristic odor.

## 12.20. Urea Cycle Defects

*For example*:
   i. Citrullinemia
   ii. Ornithine transcarbamylase deficiency
   iii. Arginosuccinic aciduria.
1. Result from the inability to detoxify nitrogen
2. Are characterized by:
   i. Severe hyperammonemia
   ii. Respiratory alkalosis
   iii. Typical onset after 24 hours of age.

## 12.21.  Disorders of Carbohydrate Metabolism

*For example*:
   i.   Galactosemia
   ii.  Hereditary fructose intolerance
   iii. Fructose 1,6-diphosphatase deficiency
   iv.  Glycogen storage diseases.
1. Are a heterogeneous group caused by
   i.   Inability to metabolize specific sugars
   ii.  Aberrant glycogen synthesis
   iii. Disorders of gluconeogenesis.
2. They may manifest with:
   i.   Hypoglycemia
   ii.  Hepatosplenomegaly
   iii. Lactic acidosis or ketosis.

## 12.22.  Lysosomal Storage Disorders

*For example*:
   i.   Mucopolysaccharidosis
   ii.  Tay-Sachs
   iii. Niemann-Pick disease
   iv.  Gaucher's disease.
1. Are caused by accumulation of glycoproteins, glycolipids, or glycosaminoglycans within lysosomes in various tissues.
2. They usually present later in infancy, not with a specific laboratory abnormality, but with:
   i.   Organomegaly
   ii.  Facial coarseness
   iii. Neurodegeneration
   iv.  Progressively degenerative course.

## 12.23.  Peroxisomal Disorders

*For example*:
   i.   Zellweger syndrome
   ii.  Neonatal adrenoleukodystrophy.
1. Result from failure of the peroxisomal enzymes.
2. They may present with features similar to the lysosomal storage disorders.
3. Common features of Zellweger syndrome include:
   i.   Large fontanel
   ii.  Organomegaly
   iii. Down-like facies
   iv.  Seizures
   v.   Chondrodysplasia punctata.

## Bibliography

1. http://emedicine.medscape.com/article/1150420-overview
2. http://ghr.nlm.nih.gov/condition/galactosemia
3. http://ghr.nlm.nih.gov/condition/phenylketonuria
4. http://pediatrics.aappublications.org/content/123/1/19
5. http://www.cdc.gov/newbornscreening
6. http://www.ucsfbenioffchildrens.org/pdf/manuals/53_Metabolism.pdf
7. http://www.ucsfbenioffchildrens.org/pdf/manuals/53_Metabolism.pdf
8. www.nccpeds.com/powerpoints/IEM_Ellefson.ppt

# Neonatology

## 13.1. Lethal Neonatal Dwarfism

### 13.1.1. Usually fatal

- Achondrogenesis (different types)
- Campomelic dysplasia
- Chondrodysplasia punctata (rhizomelic form)
- Dyssegmental dysplasia, Silverman-Handmaker type
- Short rib polydactyly, Majewski type, Saldino-Noonan type
- Homozygous achondroplasia
- Hypophosphatasia (congenital form)
- Osteopetrosis (congenital form)
- Osteogenesis imperfecta, type II
- Thanatophoric dysplasia.

### 13.1.2. Often fatal

Asphyxiating thoracic dystrophy (Jeune syndrome).

### 13.1.3. Occasionally fatal

- Ellis-van Creveld syndrome
- Diastrophic dysplasia
- Metatropic dwarfism
- Kniest dysplasia.

## 13.2. Usually Nonlethal Dwarfing Conditions

Recognizable at birth or within first new months of life.

### 13.2.1. Most common

- Achondroplasia
- Diastrophic dysplasia
- Spondyloepiphyseal dysplasia congenita

- Osteogenesis imperfecta (types I, III, and IV)
- Ellis-van Creveld syndrome.

### 13.2.2. Less common

- Chondrodysplasia punctata (some forms)
- Kniest dysplasia (not severe congenital forms)
- Metatropic dysplasia
- Langer mesomelic dysplasia.

## 13.3. Incidence of Malformation and Degree of Maternal Hyperglycemia Prior to Conception

Mothers should keep:
1. Fasting blood sugars at 60–100 mg/dL.
2. Keep 1-hour postmeal values at 100–140 mg/dL.
3. Before diabetic women become pregnant, they should have glycosylated hemoglobin (HbA1c) of < 6% and it should be maintained during pregnancy.

## 13.4. Known Risk Factors for Prematurity Include

1. Placenta bleeding (placenta previa, abruptio placentae)
2. Bacterial vaginosis
3. Uterine abnormalities (bicornuate uterus, incompetent cervix)
4. Congenital abnormalities
5. Cocaine abuse
6. Polyhydramnios
7. Maternal chronic diseases
8. Group B streptococcus (GBS)
9. Premature rapture of membranes (PROM)
10. Sexually transmitted diseases (herpes and syphilis)
11. Chorioamnionitis
12. Periodontal diseases.

## 13.5. Independent Risk Factors for Increased Mortality among Preterm Infants

| | |
|---|---|
| Male sex | Persistent bradycardia at 5 minutes |
| 5-minute Apgar < 4 | Hypothermia |
| Lack of antenatal steroids | Intrauterine growth restriction (IUGR) |

## 13.6.  Algorithm for Management of Baby Born to Mom with Group B Streptococcus Infection (GBS) Prophylaxis

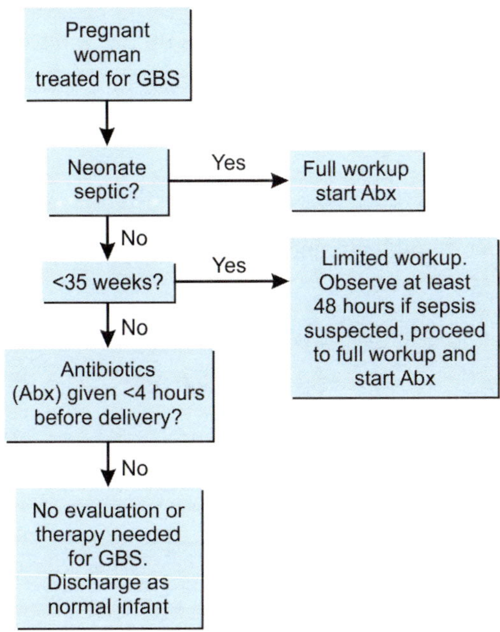


## 13.7.  Apgar Score (After Virginia Apgar)

**A:**  Activity (muscle tone)

**P:**  Pulse (heart rate)

**G:**  Grimace (reflex irritability)

**A:**  Appearance (color)

**R:**  Respiration.

### 13.7.1. Apgar score elements

| Score | 0 | 1 | 2 |
|---|---|---|---|
| Heart rate | Absent | <100 beats/minute | >100 beats/minute |
| Respiration | Absent | Slow and irregular | Good and crying |
| Muscle tone | Limp | Some flexion | Active motion |
| Reflex irritability | No response | Grimace | Cough, sneeze and cry |
| Color | Blue and pale | Body pink and blue limbs | Completely pink |

- Reflex irritability is tested in response to a catheter placed in infant's nose.
- Scoring is done at 1 minute, 5 minutes.
- Maximum score is 10.
- Score at 15 minutes <3 has been associated with >50% mortality and >60% permanent, severe neurologic sequelae in infant who survive.

## 13.8. The Used Endotracheal Tube (i.e. diameter) Based on Body Weight

### 13.8.1. The size

- <1.5 kg wt : 2.5 mm tube diameter
- – 2.5 kg wt : 3 mm diameter
- >2.5 kg wt : 3.5 mm diameter.

### 13.8.2. The length

- 1 kg wt  : 7 cm tube length
- 2 kg wt  : 8 cm tube length
- 3 kg wt  : 9 cm tube length
- 4 kg wt  : 10 cm tube length.

## 13.9. A "White Pupillary Reflex" is Abnormal, so Think of

1. Retinoblastoma
2. Retinal coloboma
3. Chorioretinitis
4. Retinopathy of prematurity.

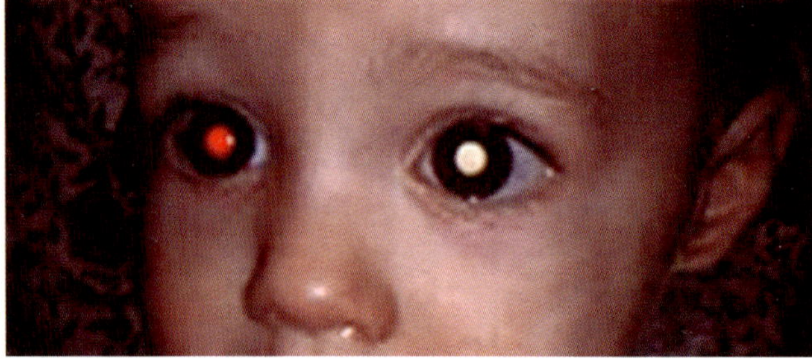

**Fig. 13.1**: White pupillary reflex

## 13.10.  Prechtl States of Sleep and Wakefulness in the Newborn

| State | Findings |
|---|---|
| 1 | Eyes closed, regular respiration and no movements |
| 2 | Eyes closed, irregular respiration and no gross movements |
| 3 | Eyes open and no gross movements |
| 4 | Eyes open, gross movements and no cry |
| 5 | Crying and eyes can be open or closed |

## 13.11.  Glucose Screening

- Routine glucose screening is no longer recommended.

### 13.11.1. Screening should be directed toward those infants at risk for pathologic hypoglycemia

| | |
|---|---|
| Born to mother with diabetes | Low birth weight (<2,500 gm) |
| Large for gestational age (LGA) | Polycythemia (HCT > 70%) |
| Small for gestational age (SGA) | Hypothermia |
| Premature (< 37 weeks gestation) | Low APGAR scores (<5 at 1 minute) |
| Stress (sepsis, respiratory distress and other abnormalities) | |

### 13.11.2. Screen if any of these clinical signs are noted

| | |
|---|---|
| Tremors and irritability | Cyanosis, apnea and tachypnea |
| High-pitched cry | Poor suck |
| Lethargy and hypotonia | Jitteriness |
| Seizures | |

## 13.12. The "Primitive" Reflexes

1. **Moro reflex:**
   Hold the baby up off the bed by its hands in abduction, lift its shoulders a few inches off the bed and then release the baby's hands
   So: The normal response is for the baby to rapidly abduct and extend its arms, followed by complete opening of the hands.
2. **Finger grasp:**
   Insert your fingers in to the baby's hands to get flexion of its fingers around your fingers then lift the baby while he/she holds on to your fingers with his/her palmar grasp.
3. **Automatic walking (stepping reflex):**
   Hold the baby upright with its feet on the table/bed in a standing position, then tilt the baby slightly forward
   So: The baby should make a step forward.
4. **Suck–swallow reflex:**
   Place your finger in the baby's mouth and note the strength and rhythm of sucking and its synchrony with swallowing.

## 13.13. The Clinical Problems Associated with Small for Gestational Age (SGA) at Birth

| Asphyxia | |
|---|---|
| Temperature instability | Metabolic abnormalities (both protein and lipid) |
| Glucose abnormalities (both hypo- and hyper-) | Neurodevelopmental abnormalities |
| Immune dysfunction | Polycythemia—Hyperviscosity |

## 13.14. Complications of Diabetes in Pregnancy on the Fetuses and Infants

Infants of mothers with gestational diabetes only (onset only in pregnancy) are at increased risk for all of the followings except for congenital abnormalities and future obesity/diabetes:

| | |
|---|---|
| Sudden fetal death in the 3rd trimester | Cardiomyopathy |
| Macrosomia | Congenital heart disease |
| Increased rate of C-section | Septal defects |
| IUGR | Transposition of great arteries |
| Hypoglycemia | Truncus arteriosus |
| Hypocalcemia | Coarctation |
| Hypomagnesemia | Unconjugated hyperbilirubinemia |
| Polycythemia | Small left-colon syndrome |
| Renal anomalies | |

### 13.15. The Risk of Developing Respiratory Distress Syndrome (RDS) Hyaline Membrane Disease (HMD) is

### 13.15.1. The risk increased by the following factors

- Premature birth
- Male gender
- Hypothermia
- Fetal distress/asphyxia
- Caucasian race
- C-section
- Diabetic mother
- Second-born twin
- Family history of HMD.

### 13.15.2. Reduced by the following factors

- Maternal hypertension
- Premature rapture of membranes
- Subacute placental abruption
- Maternal use of narcotics.

### 13.16. Persistent Pulmonary Hypertension of the Newborn (PPHN)—The Most Commonly Identified Etiologies

1. Meconium aspiration
2. Pulmonary infections
3. HMD
4. Sepsis
5. Pulmonary hypoplasia
6. Hyperviscosity/polycythemia
7. Hypoglycemia
8. Hypothermia.

### 13.17. Do Not Use Indomethacin in Treatment of Patent Ductus Arteriosus (PDA) if the Infant has Any of the Following

- Necrotizing enterocolitis
- Serum creatinine >1.6 mg/dL
- Hourly urine output<1 mL/kg
- Bleeding diathesis
- Platelets <50,000.

### 13.17.1. Note:

1.  It is OK to use if the infant has an interventricular hemorrhage.
2.  Indomethacin loses its effectiveness fairly quickly.
3.  By 3–4 days, it is less effective because of prostaglandins play a less significant role in keeping PDA open.

## 13.18.  Meconium Plugs Occur More Commonly in Infants with

- Small left colon syndrome
- Cystic fibrosis (CF)
- Hypothyroidism
- Rectal aganglionosis
- Maternal drug abuse
- Magnesium sulfate therapy for pre-eclampsia.

## 13.19.  Risk Factors for Severe Hyperbilirubinemia

- Predischarge total bilirubin in a high-risk zone defined as >95th percentile for age.
- Jaundice within the first 24 hours of life.
- Hemolytic disease due to immune- mediated hemolysis.
- Gestational age 35–36 weeks.
- Previous sibling who required phototherapy.
- Cephalhematoma.
- Significant bruising from birth trauma.
- An infant who is exclusively breast- fed and lost >12% of body weight.
- East-Asian or Greek race.

### 13.19.1.  Other minor risk factors include

- Gestational age ≥ 41 weeks
- African-American race
- Male gender.

## 13.20.  Neonatal Jaundice

### 13.20.1. Jaundice appears after the 3rd day during the first week suggests

- Sepsis
- Urinary tract infections
- Congenital infection (syphilis and CMV).

## 13.20.2. Jaundice occurs after the first week considers

- Breast milk jaundice
- Sepsis
- Galactosemia
- Hypothyroidism
- CF
- Congenital atresia of the biliary ducts
- Hepatitis
- Spherocytosis
- Other weird hemolytic anemia, e.g. pyruvate kinase deficiency
- Drugs (specially in G6PD deficiency).

## 13.20.3. Jaundice is persistent, so think of the following

- Inspissated bile syndrome
- Hyperalimentation/drug-induced cholestasis
- Hepatitis
- A TORCH disease
- Congenital atresia of the bile ducts
- Galactosemia.

## 13.21. Guidelines for Implementing Phototherapy in Hyperbilirubinemia

### 13.21.1. For infants at low-risk

($\geq$ 38 weeks gestation and without risk factors)
Phototherapy is started at the following total serum bilirubin values:
- 24 hours of age: > 12 mg/dL (205 mmol/L)
- 48 hours of age: > 15 mg/dL (257 mmol/L)
- 72 hours of age: > 18 mg/dL (308 mmol/L).

### 13.21.2. For infants at medium risk

($\geq$ 38 weeks gestation with risk factors or 35–37 6/7 weeks without risk factors)
Phototherapy is started at the following total serum bilirubin values:
- 24 hours of age: > 10 mg/dL (171 mmol/L)
- 48 hours of age: > 13 mg/dL (222 mmol/L)
- 72 hours of age: > 15 mg/dL (257 mmol/L).

### 13.21.3. For infants at high-risk

(35–37 6/7 weeks with risk factors)
Phototherapy is started at the following total serum bilirubin values:
- 24 hours of age: > 8 mg/dL (137 mmol/L)
- 48 hours of age: > 11 mg/dL (188 mmol/L)
- 72 hours of age: > 13.5 mg/dL (231 mmol/L).

### 13.21.4. Risk factors

- Isoimmune hemolytic disease
- Glucose-6-phosphate dehydrogenase (G6PD)deficiency
- Asphyxia
- Significant lethargy
- Temperature instability
- Sepsis
- Acidosis
- Albumin <3.0 gm/dL.

## 13.22. Guidelines for Implementing Exchange Transfusion in Hyperbilirubinemia

### 13.22.1. For infants at low-risk

(≥ 38 weeks gestation and without risk factors)
Exchange transfusion is indicated for the following total serum bilirubin values:
- 24 hours of age: > 19 mg/dL (325 mmol/L)
- 48 hours of age: > 22 mg/dL (376 mmol/L)
- 72 hours of age: > 24 mg/dL (410 mmol/L)
- Any age: ≥ 25 mg/dL (428 mmol/L).

### 13.22.2. For infants at medium risk

(≥ 38 weeks gestation with risk factors or 35–37 6/7 weeks without risk factors)
Exchange transfusion is indicated for the following total serum bilirubin values:
- 24 hours of age: > 16.5 mg/dL (282 mmol/L)
- 48 hours of age: > 19 mg/dL (325 mmol/L)
- ≥ 72 hours of age: > 21 mg/dL (359 mmol/L).

### 13.22.3. For infants at high-risk

(35–37 6/7 weeks with risk factors)
Exchange transfusion is indicated for the following total serum bilirubin values:
- 24 hours of age: > 15 mg/dL (257 mmol/L)

- 48 hours of age: > 17 mg/dL (291 mmol/L)
- ≥ 72 hours of age: > 18.5 mg/dL (316 mmol/L).

## 13.23.  Congenital Syphilis

If an infant is born to a mother with a +VDRL or +RPR, examine the infant for clinical findings of congenital syphilis:
- Nonimmune hydrops
- Jaundice
- Hepatosplenomegaly
- Rhinitis
- Pseudoparalysis of an extremity
- Skin rash:
    1.   Vesicular lesions
    2.   Vesiculobullous lesions
    3.   Superficial desquamation.
- Uveitis /chorioretinitis.

## 13.24.  Neonatal Seizures

### 13.24. 1.  Causes of neonatal seizures

#### 13.24.1.1. Age 1–4 days

- Hypoxic-ischemic encephalopathy
- Drug withdrawal, maternal drug use of narcotic or barbiturates
- Drug toxicity: lidocaine and penicillin
- Intraventricular hemorrhage
- Acute metabolic disorders:
    1.   IIypocalccmia
    2.   Hypoglycemia
    3.   Hypomagnesemia
    4.   Hyponatremia or hypernatremia
- Inborn errors of metabolism
    1.   Galactosemia
    2.   Hyperglycinemia
    3.   Urea cycle disorders
- Pyridoxine deficiency.

#### 13.24.1.2. Age 4–14 days

- Infection.
- Metabolic disorders.

- Drug withdrawal, maternal drug use of narcotic or barbiturates.
- Benign neonatal convulsions, familial and nonfamilial.
- Kernicterus and hyperbilirubinemia.
- Developmental delay, epilepsy and neonatal diabetes (DEND) syndrome.

### 13.24.1.3. Age 2–8 weeks

- Infection
- Head injury
- Inherited disorders of metabolism
- Malformations of cortical development
- Tuberous sclerosis
- Sturge-Weber syndrome.

## 13.24.2. Facts about neonatal seizures

### 13.24.2.1. Definition

Neonatal seizures, as with any other type of seizure, are paroxysmal, repetitive and stereotypical events.

### 13.24.2.2. Presentation

1. They are usually clinically subtle, inconspicuous and difficult to recognize from the normal behaviors of the interictal periods or physiological phenomena.
2. There is no recognizable postictal state.
3. Generalized tonic clonic seizures (GTCS) are exceptional.

### 13.24.2.3. Main types of neonatal seizures

The most widely used scheme is by Volpe of five main types of neonatal seizure:
- Subtle seizures (50%)
- Tonic seizures (5%)
- Clonic seizures (25%)
- Myoclonic seizures (20%)
- Nonparoxysmal repetitive behaviors.

## 13.25. Characteristic Features of Early- and Late-onset Neonatal Listerosis

| Early onset (< 5 days) | Late onset (≥ 5 days) |
|---|---|
| Positive result of maternal Listeria culture | Negative results of maternal Listeria culture |
| Obstetric complications | Uncomplicated pregnancy |
| Premature delivery | Term delivery |
| Low birth weight | Normal birth weight |
| Neonatal sepsis | Neonatal meningitis |
| Mean age at onset 1.5 days | Mean age at onset 14.2 days |
| Mortality rate is >30% | Mortality rate is <10% |

## 13.26. Characteristic Features of Early- and Late-onset GBS Disease

| | Early-onset disease | Late-onset disease |
|---|---|---|
| Age at onset | 0–6 days | 7–90 days |
| Increased risk after obstetric complications | Yes | No |
| Common clinical manifestations | Sepsis, pneumonia and meningitis | Bacteremia, meningitis and other focal infections |
| Common serotypes | Ia, III, V, II, Ib | III predominates |
| Case fatality rate | 4.7% | 2.8% |

## 13.27. Screening for Inborn Errors of Metabolism that Cause Neonatal Seizures

### 13.27.1. Blood glucose low

- Fructose 1,6-diphosphatase deficiency
- Glycogen storage disease type I
- Maple syrup urine disease.

### 13.27.2. Blood calcium low

- Hypoparathyroidism
- Maternal hyperparathyroidism.

### 13.27.3. Blood ammonia high

- Argininosuccinic acidemia
- Carbamylphosphate synthetase deficiency
- Citrullinemia
- Methylmalonic acidemia (may be normal)
- Multiple carboxylase deficiency
- Ornithine transcarbamylase deficiency
- Propionic acidemia (may be normal).

### 13.27.4. Blood lactate high

- Fructose 1,6-diphosphatase deficiency
- Glycogen storage disease type I
- Mitochondrial disorders
- Multiple carboxylase deficiency.

### 13.27.5. Metabolic acidosis

- Fructose 1,6-diphosphatase deficiency
- Glycogen storage disease type I
- Maple syrup urine disease
- Methylmalonic acidemia
- Multiple carboxylase deficiency
- Propionic acidemia.

## 13.28.  Pathophysiology of Meconium Passage and the Meconium Aspiration Syndrome

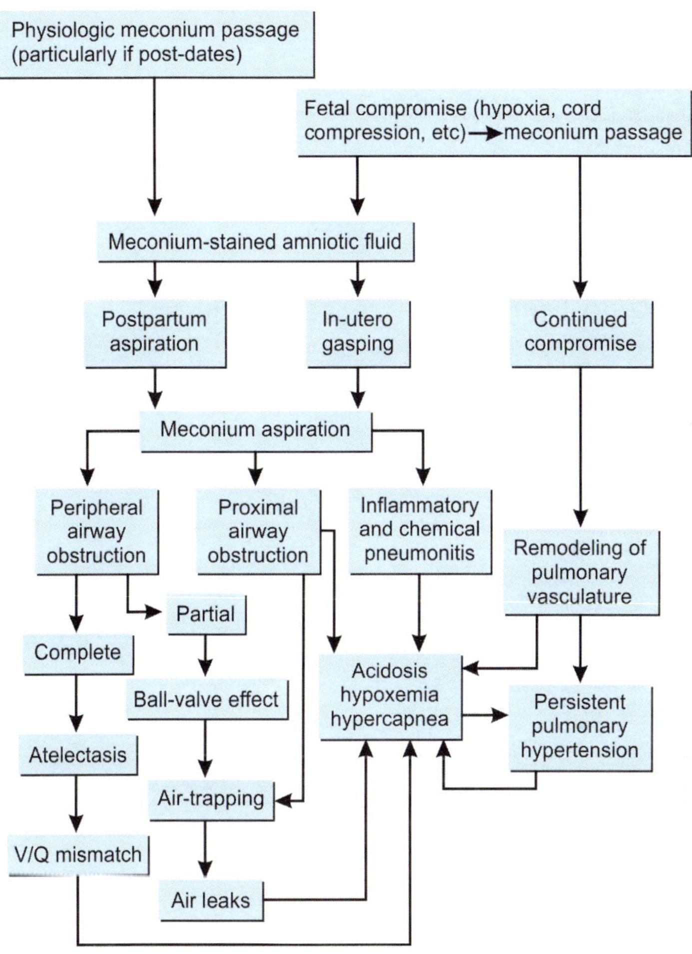


## 13.29.  Congenital Infections

### 13.29.1. Features of congenital Cytomegalovirus infection

1.  Small for dates
2.  Mental retardation
3.  Petechial rash
4.  Seizures
5.  Hepatosplenomegaly
6.  Central nervous system calcification
7.  Chorioretinitis

8.  Microgyria
9.  Deafness.

## 13.29.2. Features of congenital rubella infection

1.  Growth retardation
2.  Cataracts
3.  Purpura
4.  Deafness
5.  Thrombocytopenia
6.  Perivascular necrotic areas
7.  Hepatosplenomegaly
8.  Polymicrogyria
9.  Congenital heart disease
10.  Heterotopias
11.  Chorioretinitis
12.  Subependymal cavitations.

## 13.29.3. Features of congenital toxoplasmosis infection

1.  Purpura
2.  Hydrocephalus
3.  Hepatosplenomegaly
4.  Chorioretinitis
5.  Jaundice
6.  Cerebral calcification
7.  Convulsions.

## 13.30.  Neonatal Features of Maternal Drugs Intake Prenatally

### 13.30.1. Fetal alcohol syndrome

1.  Growth retardation
2.  Feeding problems
3.  Ptosis
4.  Neuroglial heterotopia
5.  Absent philtrum and hypoplastic upper lip
6.  Disorganization of neurons
7.  Congenital heart disease.

### 13.30.2. Fetal phenytoin syndrome

1.  Growth delay
2.  Broad nasal ridge
3.  Hypoplasia of distal phalanges
4.  Anteverted nostrils
5.  Inner epicanthic folds.

## 13.31.  Definitions by World Health Organization (WHO)

### 13.31.1. Gestation (independent of birth weight)

1.  Preterm = Less than 37 completed weeks of gestation (258 days).
2.  Full-term = Between 37 weeks and 42 completed weeks of gestation (259–293 days).
3.  Post-term or postmature = More than 42 completed weeks (294 days).

Dates are taken from the first day of the last menstrual period.

### 13.31.2. Birth weight (independent of gestation)

1.  Low birth weight = Less than 2500 gm
2.  Very low birth weight = Less than 1500 gm (accepted by convention)
3.  Extremely low birth weight = Less than 1000 gm
4.  Impossibly or incredibly low birth weight =  Less than 750 gm.

### 13.31.3. Size for gestation

1.  Small for gestation (SGA) = Less than 10th centile in weight expected for gestation (small for dates).
2.  Appropriate for gestation (AGA) = Between 10th and 90th centiles of weight expected for gestation.
3.  Large for gestation (LGA) = More than 90th centile in weight expected for gestation.

### 13.31.4. The neonate

1.  Perinatal period = The period from 24 weeks' gestation or the time of the live birth if less than 24 weeks' gestation, to 7 days of postnatal age.
2.  Early neonatal period = The first 7 days of life of a liveborn infant of any gestation.
3.  Late neonatal period = 8–28 days after birth.
4.  Neonatal period = The first 28 days of life of a liveborn infant of any gestation.
5.  Infancy = The first year of life.

### 13.31.5. Mortality rates

1.  Stillbirth rate = Number of stillbirths per 1000 total births.
2.  Perinatal mortality rate (PMR) = Number of stillbirths + early (upto 7 days) neonatal deaths per1000 total births.
3.  Neonatal mortality rate (NNMR) = Number of deaths in the first 28 days per 1000 live births.
4.  Infant mortality rate (IMR) = Number of deaths in the first 365 days per 1000 live births.

## 13.32.  Conditions Predisposing to Birth Injury

| | |
|---|---|
| Poor maternal health | Cephalopelvic disproportion |
| Maternal age (very young and old) | Hydrocephalus |
| Grand multiparity | Macrosomia |
| Twins (particularly the second) | Dystocia |
| Prematurity/low birth weight | Contracted pelvis |
| Malpresentation | Instrumental delivery |

## 13.33.  The Major Clinical Features for Grading the Severity of Hypoxic-Ischemic Encephalopathy

| Mild | Moderate | Severe |
|---|---|---|
| Irritability | Lethargy | Coma |
| Hyper-alert | Seizures | Prolonged seizures |
| Normal tone | Differential tone (legs > arms) (neck extensors > flexors) | Severe hypotonia |
| Weak suck | Poor suck and requires tubefeeds | No sucking reflex |
| Sympathetic dominance | Parasympathetic dominance | Coma and requires respiratory support |

## 13.34.  Differential Diagnosis for Hypoxic-Ischemic Encephalopathy

| Condition | Examples |
|---|---|
| Infective | • Meningitis (bacterial or viral)<br>• Encephalitis (herpes simplex) |
| Traumatic brain lesion | • Subdural hemorrhage |
| Vascular | • Neonatal stroke<br>• Shock secondary to acute blood loss (antepartum/intrapartum) |
| Metabolic | • Hypoglycemia<br>• Hypo/hypernatremia<br>• Bilirubin encephalopathy |
| Inborn error of metabolism | • Urea cycle defects<br>• Pyridoxine dependency<br>• Lactate acidemias<br>• Aminoacidemias<br>• Organic acidemias |
| Congenital brain malformation | • Neuronal migration disorder |
| Neuromuscular disorder | • Spinal muscular atrophy |
| Maternal drug exposure | • Acute or chronic |

### 13.35. Etiology of the Small for Gestational Age (SGA) Neonate

| Maternal causes | |
| --- | --- |
| These consist of in utero starvation and placental insufficiency | |
| • Essential hypertension | • Multiple pregnancy |
| • Pregnancy-associated hypertension (PET) | • Poor socioeconomic circumstances with severe malnutrition |
| • Chronic renal disease | • Excess smoking |
| • Long-standing diabetes | • Excess alcohol |
| • Heart disease in pregnancy | • Living at high altitude |
| **Fetal causes** | |
| Congenital abnormality (chromosomal and many syndromes, e.g. potter) | Congenital infection (rubella, toxoplasmosis, cytomegalovirus, herpes simplex and syphilis) | Early fetal toxins such as alcohol, phenytoin and warfarin |

### 13.36. Problems of the Small for Gestational Age (SGA) Neonate

- Hypoglycemia.
- Hypothermia.
- Polycythemia.
- Neutropenia and thrombocytopenia.
- Hypocalcemia.
- Infection.
- Congenital abnormality (3–6%).
- Pulmonary hemorrhage.
- Other humoral and metabolic abnormalities (high ammonia, urea, and uric acid levels, high circulating cortisol, corticosterone and growth hormone levels after birth.

### 13.37. Etiology of the Large for Gestational Age (LGA) Neonate

1. Constitutionally large baby from heavy large mother.
2. Maternal diabetes or prediabetes—The infant of the diabetic mother (IDM) or the infant of the gestational diabetic mother (IGDM).
3. Severe erythroblastosis.
4. Other causes of hydrops fetalis and ascites.
5. Transposition of the great arteries (sometimes).
6. Syndromes:
   a. Beckwith-Wiedemann (BW) syndrome
   b. Sotos syndrome
   c. Marshall syndrome
   d. Weaver syndrome.

### 13.38. Problems of the Large for Gestational Age (LGA) Neonate

- Birth asphyxia and trauma
- Hypoglycemia
- Polycythemia
- Apparent large postnatal weight loss.

### 13.39. Complications of Parenteral Nutrition

1. Catheter related
   a. Sepsis-bacterial or fungal
   b. Thrombosis/obstruction
   c. Hemorrhage
   d. Extravasation of fluid from peripheral lines
   e. Catheter displacement and breakage or removal.
2. Metabolic related
   a. Cholestasis—Often reversible, and reduced by minimal enteral feeding.
   b. Fat embolism and lipid overload—Rare.
   c. Hyperglycemia and glycosuria.
   d. Hyperammonemia and acidosis—Rare.

### 13.40. Factors Affecting the Incidence of RDS

| Decrease | Increase |
| --- | --- |
| Intrauterine growth retardation | Asphyxia |
| Prolonged rupture of membranes | Severe rhesus disease |
| Maternal steroid therapy | Maternal diabetes |
| Maternal smoking | Maternal hypertension |
| Sickle cell disease | Antepartum hemorrhage |
| Heroin | Elective cesarean section |
| Alcohol | Second twin |
| Black infants | Family history |
| Girls | Boys |

### Bibliography


1. http://emedicine.medscape.com/article/410969-overview#a19
2. http://emedicine.medscape.com/article/898437-overview
3. http://pediatrics.aappublications.org/content/120/6/1390.full
4. http://www.cdc.gov/Features/PrematureBirth/
5. http://www.cdc.gov/groupbstrep/about/newborns-pregnant.html

6. http://www.medscape.com/medline/abstract/5063132
7. http://www.ncbi.nlm.nih.gov/books/NBK2599/
8. J. Eric Piña-Garza. Finisher's clinical pediatric neurology. Seventh edition. Saunders 2013.
9. www.kellogg.umich.edu
10. www.thenurseslockerroom.com

# Nephrology

## 14.1. Most Frequent Hereditary—Metabolic Diseases of Childhood that Lead to End-stage Renal Disease

1. Nephronophthisis-medullary cystic disease
2. Nephropathic and juvenile cystinosis
3. Congenital nephrotic syndrome
4. Primary oxalosis with oxaluria
5. Alport syndrome
6. Nail-patella syndrome
7. Polycystic kidney disease (both infantile and adult varieties).

## 14.2. Causes of End-stage Renal Disease (ESRD) Vary with the Patient's Age and Include

- Congenital renal diseases (53%)
- Glomerulonephritides (20%)
- Focal segmental glomerular sclerosis (12%)
- Metabolic diseases (10%)
- Miscellaneous (5%).

## 14.3. Causes of Anemia in Chronic Kidney Disease (CKD)

1. Abnormally low erythropoietin levels (most common)
2. Functional or absolute iron deficiency
3. Blood loss (either occult or overt)
4. Uremic inhibitors (e.g. parathyroid hormone {PTH}, spermine, etc.)
5. Reduced half-life of circulating blood cells
6. Folate deficiency
7. Vitamin $B_{12}$ deficiency
8. Combination of these with a deficiency of erythropoietin.

## 14.4. Schwartz Formula for Estimation of Creatinine Clearance

**Creatinine clearance = K × (height in cm/plasma creatinine in mg/dL)**
K is an age-dependent constant.

### 14.4.1. Creatinine clearance

- 0.45 for children <2 years
- 0.55 for children and adolescent girls
- 0.70 for adolescent boys.

## 14.5.  Important Concepts Used in Determining Acid-base Status

### 14.5.1. What effect ventilation, which is reflected in the $PaCO_2$, has on pH and $HCO_3^-$

### 14.5.2. What effect metabolic alkalosis or acidosis, reflected in the $HCO_3^-$, has on $PaCO_2$ (ventilation)

### 14.5.3. Anion gap and osmolal gap

Note:

    I.  Normal serum anion gap (AG) is 12

$$AG = Na^+ - (Cl^- + HCO_3^-)$$

    II.  Normal urine anion gap (UAG) is negative, indicating that kidney is producing an unmeasured cation, i.e. ammonia $(NH_4^+)$

$$UAG = Na^+ + K^+ - Cl^-$$

## 14.6.  Changes in Blood Chemistry—Respiratory vs Metabolic Disorders

| Equilibrium reactions between $PaCO_2$ and $HCO_3^-$ | | Then pH changes: (acute/ chronic) | Then $HCO_3^-$ changes: (acute/ chronic) | Then $PaCO_2$ changes: |
|---|---|---|---|---|
| Respiratory disorders | If $PaCO_2$ decreased by 10 | 0.08<br>0.04 | −2<br>−5 | |
| | If $PaCO_2$ increased by 10 | −0.08<br>−0.04 | 1<br>4 | |
| Metabolic disorders | If $HCO_3^-$ decreased by 10 | | | −12 |
| | If $HCO_3^-$ increased by 10 | | | 6 |

## 14.7.  Metabolic Acidosis

Metabolic acidosis occurs with:
- Overproduction of lactic acids or ketoacids
- $HCO_3^-$ wasting (renal tubular acidosis or diarrhea)
- Underexcreation of acid (renal failure)
- Poisoning by agents that are metabolized to acids.

Approach for evaluating metabolic acidosis

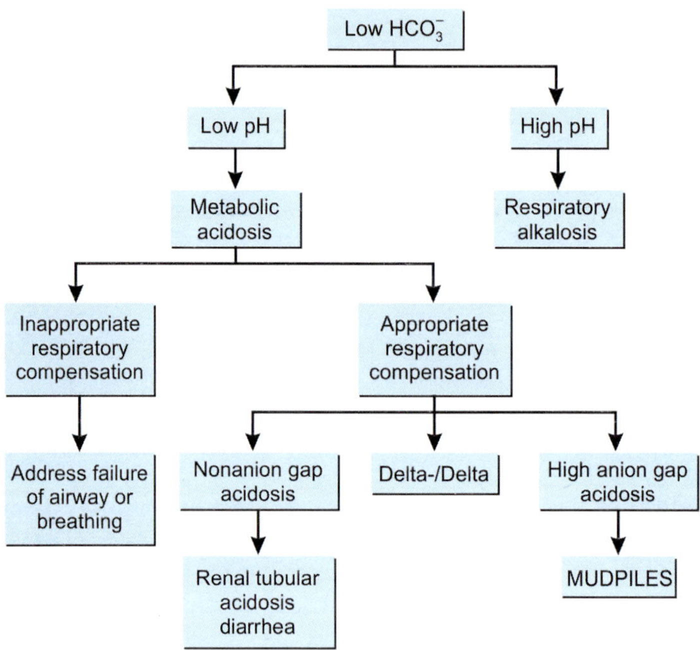


## 14.8.  Anion Gap and Metabolic Acidosis

| Causes of increased anion gap metabolic acidosis: | |
| --- | --- |
| **Causes** | **Examples** |
| 1.  Severe chronic renal failure (CRF) | Decreased acid (specially $NH_4^+$) excretion-most common |
| 2.  Ketoacidosis | Diabetes, alcoholic and starvation |
| 3.  Lactic acidosis | Drugs, toxins, circulatory compromise |
| 4.  Poisoning | Salicylates, methanol, ethylene glycol |

## 14.9.  Analysis of Acid-base Problems

### 14.9.1. First step

1.  Acidosis or alkalosis?

    Determine primary abnormality: Respiratory or metabolic (**Role 1**).

2.  Calculate anion gap (**Role 2**).

3.  If an anion gap (AG) is present, then calculate the difference between the calculated AG and a normal AG of 12.

    This is also known as Δ-Δ (delta-delta) (**Role 3**).

4.  Is there compensation?

    If $pCO_2$ and $HCO_3^-$ are changed in opposite directions, there must be more than one disorder.

### 14.9.2.  Second step

We'll go through these roles.

#### 14.9.2.1.Role 1: Look at the pH

> < 7.35 indicates acidemia
>
> > 7.45 indicates alkalemia.

#### 14.9.2.2.Role 2: Calculate the anion gap

$$AG = Na^+ - (Cl^- + HCO_3^-)$$

If the AG is ≥ 20:
- There is a primary metabolic acidosis, regardless of pH or bicarbonate
- There is an anion gap metabolic acidosis.

#### 14.9.2.3.Role 3: Calculate the excess anion gap (when Ag is increased)

Using the delta-delta, which uses:
- The differences between measured and normal anion gap
- The difference between measured and normal bicarbonate.

14.9.2.3.1. So

  i.  Find the difference between measured and normal anion gap

  ii.  Then add the measured bicarbonate

    (Measured anion gap -12) + measured bicarbonate

    The result will then be compared to normal bicarbonate.

14.9.2.3.2. If the result is:

  i.  Greater than a high-normal bicarbonate (30)

    → an underlying metabolic alkalosis.

   ii. Less than a low-normal bicarbonate (24)
      → an underlying nonanion gap metabolic acidosis.

## 14.10. Persistent Asymptomatic Hematuria

In an otherwise healthy child can usually be attributed to 1 of 4 causes:

1. Idiopathic hypercalciuria (diagnosed with urine calcium: creatinine >0.2).
2. IgA nephropathy.
3. Thin basement membrane disease.
4. Early Alport syndrome (family history of hearing loss or renal failure—specially in males).

## 14.11. Evaluation of Hematuria in Children—Tests for All Children at Initial Presentation

1. CBC
2. Urinalysis
3. Serum creatinine
4. Urine calcium: Creatinine ratio (U Ca: cr)
   Urine protein: Creatinine ratio (Upr:cr)
5. Serum $C_3$ level
6. Ultrasound (if above don't reveal the problem).

## 14.12. Evaluation of Hematuria in Children—Tests for Selected Children

### 14.12.1. Laboratory tests

- DNase B titer/streptozyme if hematuria <6 months duration
- Throat culture for group A streptococcus
- Culture of skin lesion consistent with group A streptococcus
- ANA titer
- Urine RBC morphology
- Coagulation studies
- Sickle cell screen
- ANCA test
- Anti-GBM test.

### 14.12.2. Voiding cystourethrogram

With infection or when suspicion of lower tract infection.

### 14.12.3. Renal biopsy indicated for the following

- Persistent microscopic hematuria
- Hematuria with diminished renal function
- Proteinuria exceeding 150 mg/24 hours
- Hypertension
- Recurrent episode of gross hematuria.

### 14.12.4. Cystoscopy indicated for the following

- Pink to red hematuria
- Dysuria with a sterile urine culture.

## 14.13.  Classical Features of Henoch-Schönlein Purpura (HSP) (Anaphylactoid Purpura)

1. Purpuric rash (over the buttocks, abdomen and lower extremities)
2. Abdominal pain
3. Arthralgias
4. Glomerulonephritis with IgA deposition.

## 14.14.  Classical Features of Nephrotic Syndrome Usually Includes

- Proteinuria > 50 mg/kg /24 hours (or >3.5 gm/24 hours)
- Serum albumin <3 mg/dL
- Edema
- Hypercholesterolemia.

## 14.15.  Poor Prognostic Features of Hemolytic Uremic Syndrome

- Anuria lasting longer than 2 weeks.
- Initial neutrophil count >20,000.
- Coma on admission.
- Atypical forms of the disease (e.g. the diarrheal form has a better prognosis).

## 14.16.  Facts About Renal Tubular Acidosis (RTA)

### 14.16.1. Facts concerning RTA

- All RTAs have a normal anion gap, i.e. all are hyperchloremic
- There are 3 types; one proximal (type II) and two distal (I and IV)
- There is no type III.

### 14.16.2. Facts concerning serum K$^+$, remember

- Type I is low K$^+$
- Type II is low to normal K$^+$
- Type IV is high K$^+$.

## 14.17.  Type II RTA (Proximal RTA)

### 14.17.1. Facts concerning type II RTA (proximal RTA)

- The defect is decreasing bicarbonate reabsorption in the proximal tubule.
- Caused by a mechanism similar to that of acetazolamide.
- Type II in children is frequently caused by Fanconi syndrome.
- An acidic urine (i.e. normal) is usually found in type II RTA.

### 14.17.2. Causes of type II RTA

1. Fanconi syndrome
2. Drugs (Acetazolamide and 6-mercaptopurine)
3. Heavy metal poisonings (lead, copper, mercury, cadmium)
4. Disorders of protein, carbohydrate, or amino acid metabolism
5. Multiple myeloma.

## 14.18.  Type IV RTA

### 14.18.1. Facts concerning type IV RTA

- Affects the Na$^+$/K$^+$-H$^+$ exchange mechanism in the distal tubule
- It has an effect similar to spironolactone or hypoaldosteronism
- Hyperkalemia and hyperchloremic (i.e. normal anion gap) acidosis.

### 14.18.2. Causes of type IV RTA

1. Obstructive uropathy
2. Interstitial renal disease
3. Multicystic dysplastic kidneys
4. Type I pseudohypoaldosteronism
5. Diabetic nephropathy
6. 21-hydroxylase deficiency
7. Renal transplant.

## 14.19.  Type I RTA (Distal RTA)

### 14.19.1. Facts concerning type I RTA

- Defect is only in $H^+$ secretion.
- Patient becomes acidotic and hypokalemic.
- Commonly causes renal stone (from decreased citrate excretion and hypercalciuria).

### 14.19.2. Causes of type I RTA

1. Amphotericin B
2. Toluene (glue sniffing)
3. Lithium
4. SLE
5. Sjögren's disease
6. Chronic active hepatitis.

## 14.20.  Acute Renal Failure

**N.B.** Prerenal failure is always due to a decrease in renal blood flow.

### 14.20.1. Facts concerning acute renal failure

- Fractional excretion of $Na^+$ (FE $Na^+$) is best first test in assessing renal failure
    - This is very low (<1%) in prerenal azotemia.
- Urine sediment and protein further differentiate between prerenal and acute glomerulonephritis.

If a patient has renal failure with a FE $Na^+$ <1 and a normal urine sediment (or just granular or hyaline casts), the patient has prerenal azotemia.

### 14.20.2. Prerenal causes of acute renal failure

- Severe intravascular volume loss
- Renal artery stenosis
- Congestive heart failure
- Cirrhosis of the liver
- Nephrotic syndrome
- Drugs:
    1. Diuretics (most common)
    2. NSAIDs
    3. ACE inhibitors
    4. Interleukin-2.

### 14.20.3. Intrarenal causes of acute renal failure

- Acute tubular necrosis (ATN-ischemia or nephrotoxic).
- Vascular problems (large blood vessels).
- Glomerular damage (i.e. the acute glomerular nephritides) (This is the first cause of acute renal failure in children).
- Acute interstitial nephritis.

### 14.20.4. Postrenal causes of acute renal failure

- Usually due to bladder outlet obstruction (posterior urethral valves).
- BUN: Cr ratio is elevated (because the urea diffuse back into the system).
- $K^+$ may be elevated (due to associated Type IV RTA).

## 14.21.  Causes of Chronic Interstitial Nephritis

- Renal outlet obstruction
- Drugs: Chronic analgesic abuse, cisplatin, cyclosporine
- Heavy metal (lead, cadmium)
- Sjögren's disease
- Sickle-cell disease.

## 14.22.  Risk Factors Associated with the Development of UTI

Risk factors associated with the development of UTI:
1. Age and sex
2. Race
3. Family history
4. Constipation
5. Sexual activity
6. Bladder catheterization
7. Abnormalities of the urinary tract
   - Vesicoureteric reflux (VUR)
   - Obstruction.

## 14.23.  Effects of Constipation on Urinary System

Constipation in children increases the likelihood of:
1. Urinary incontinence
2. Dysfunctional voiding
3. Large capacity
4. Poorly emptying bladder
5. UTI.

## 14.24. Differential Diagnosis of Enuresis

Differential diagnosis of enuresis
1. Urinary tract infection
2. Detrusor instability
3. Neuropathic bladder
4. Ectopic ureter
5. Posterior urethral valves
6. Chronic renal disease
7. Diabetes mellitus.

## 14.25. VUR Grading

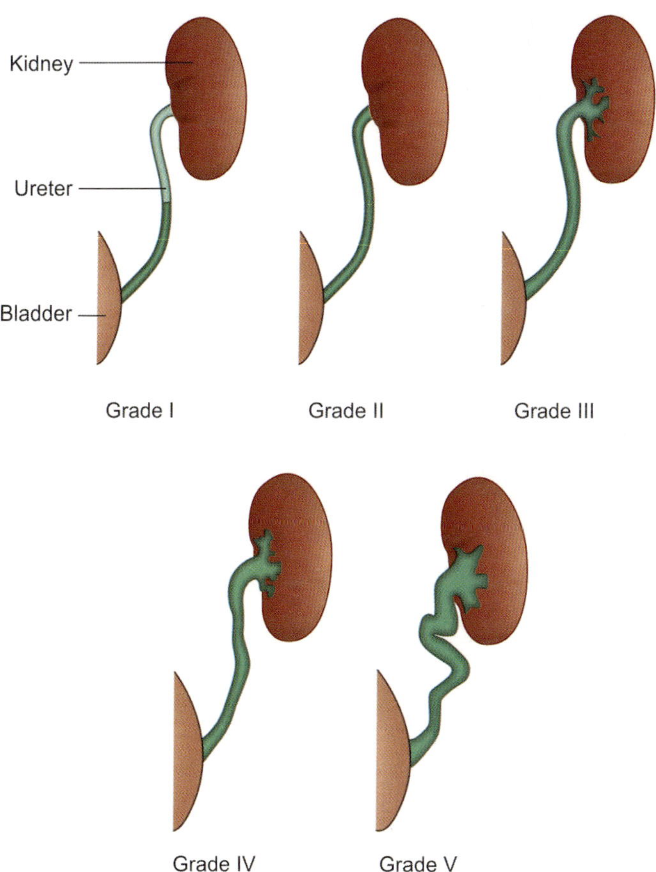


**Fig. 14.1**: VUR grading

## 14.26.  Causes of Hematuria

Causes of hematuria

1.  Infection
    a. Bacterial
    b. Viral
    c. Schistosomiasis
    d. Tuberculosis.
2.  Glomerular diseases
3.  Stones
    a. Urolithiasis
    b. Idiopathic hypercalciuria.
4.  Trauma
5.  Anatomic abnormalities
    a. Congenital abnormalities, e.g. pelviureteric junction obstruction
    b. Polycystic kidneys
    c. Tumor.
6.  Vascular
    a. Arteritis
    b. Infarction and thrombosis
    c. Loin pain—Hematuria syndrome.
7.  Hematological
    a. Coagulopathies
    b. Sickle-cell disease.
8.  Drugs, e.g. cyclophosphamide
9.  Exercise-induced
10.  Factitious.

## 14.27.  Investigations for Children with Renal Calculi

Investigations for children with renal calculi

1.  Urinalysis including pH and urine for amino acids.
2.  Urine culture.
3.  Plasma biochemistry including creatinine, chloride, bicarbonate, calcium, phosphate, urate, magnesium levels.
4.  Second morning urine sample for calcium :creatinine and oxalate: creatinine ratios (24 hours urine collections to confirm hypercalciuria or hyperoxaluria in older children).
5.  Analysis of calculus if available.

## 14.28.  Classification of Glomerular Disorders

### 14.28.1. Primary glomerulonephritis

1. Immune complex glomerulonephritis
    a. Postinfectious acute glomerulonephritis
    b. IgA nephropathy (Berger disease)
    c. Membranoproliferative glomerulonephritis (types I to III)
    d. Membranous glomerulonephritis (idiopathic).
2. Anti-GBM-antibody-mediated glomerulonephritis.
3. Uncertain etiology, e.g. minimal lesion glomerulonephritis, focal segmental glomerulosclerosis.

### 14.28.2. Glomerulonephritis associated with systemic disorders

1. Immunologically-mediated
    a. Henoch-Schönlein purpura.
    b. Systemic lupus erythematosus and other collagen disorders, e.g. scleroderma.
    c. Polyarteritis nodosa, Wegener's granulomatosis and other vasculitides.
    d. Mixed cryoglobulinemia.
    e. Systemic infections (subacute bacterial endocarditis, shunt nephritis, syphilis, malaria, hepatitis B, HIV).
2. Hereditary disorders
    a. Familial nephritis, e.g. Alport syndrome
    b. Sickle cell anemia.
3. Other conditions
    a. Diabetes mellitus
    b. Amyloidosis.

## 14.29.  Causes of Proteinuria

### 14.29.1. Intermittent proteinuria

1. Postural (orthostatic)
2. Nonpostural
    a. Exercise
    b. Fever
    c. Anatomic abnormalities, e.g. urinary tract
    d. Glomerular lesions, e.g. IgA nephropathy
    e. Random finding; no known cause.

### 14.29.2. Persistent proteinuria

1.  Glomerular
    a.  Isolated asymptomatic proteinuria.
    b.  Damage to glomerular basement membrane, e.g. acute or chronic glomerulonephritis.
    c.  Loss or reduction of basement membrane anionic charge, e.g. minimal change and congenital nephrosis.
    d.  Increased permeability in residual nephrons, e.g. chronic renal failure.
2.  Tubular
    a.  Hereditary, e.g. cystinosis, Wilson disease, Lowe syndrome, proximal tubular acidosis, galactosemia.
    b.  Acquired, e.g. interstitial nephritis, acute tubular necrosis, postrenal transplantation, pyelonephritis, vitamin D intoxication, penicillamine, heavy metal poisoning (gold, lead, mercury, etc.), analgesic abuse, drugs.

## 14.30. The Features of Nephrotic Syndrome

1.  Heavy proteinuria (> 40 mg/hour/m$^2$ or protein/creatinine ratio > 200 mg/mmol).
2.  Hypoalbuminemia (< 25 gm/L).
3.  Edema.

## 14.31. Indications for Renal Biopsy in Children with Nephrotic Syndrome

### 14.31.1. Renal biopsy is recommended before treatment with corticosteroids when the nephrotic syndrome occurs

1.  Onset at less than 6 months of age (congenital nephrotic syndrome types).
2.  Evidence of a mixed nephritic/nephrotic picture with hypertension and/or low plasma $C_3$ (pathology other than MCD more likely).

### 14.31.2. Renal biopsy may be considered in children with nephrotic syndrome

1.  Onset between 6 and 12 months of age
2.  Onset over 12 years of age (other pathology may be more likely)
3.  Persistent hypertension, microscopic hematuria, or low plasma $C_3$
4.  Renal failure—Persistent and not attributable to hypovolemia.

## 14.32.  Causes of Infantile Nephrotic Syndrome

### 14.32.1. Primary causes

a.  Congenital nephrotic syndrome—NPHS1; NPHS2 mutations.
b.  Diffuse mesangial sclerosis.
c.  Minimal change nephrotic syndrome.
d.  Focal segmental glomerulosclerosis.
e.  Denys-Drash syndrome.
f.  Nail-patella syndrome; Pierson syndrome; Galloway-Mowatt syndrome.

### 14.32.2. Secondary causes

a.  Syphilis
b.  Toxoplasmosis
c.  Cytomegalovirus
d.  Mercury
e.  Hodgkin's lymphoma or T cell malignancies.

## 14.33. Causes of Hypertension

### 14.33.1. Causes of hypertension in newborn

1.  Renal artery thrombosis
2.  Renal artery stenosis
3.  Renal venous thrombosis
4.  Congenital renal abnormalities
5.  Coarctation of the aorta
6.  Bronchopulmonary dysplasia
7.  Patent ductus arteriosus
8.  Intraventricular hemorrhage.

### 14.33.2. Causes of hypertension in the first year

1.  Coarctation of the aorta
2.  Renovascular disease
3.  Renal parenchymal diseases.

### 14.33.3. Causes of hypertension 1–6 years

1.  Renal parenchymal diseases
2.  Renovascular disease
3.  Coarctation of the aorta
4.  Endocrine causes
5.  Essential hypertension.

### 14.33.4. Causes of hypertension 6–12 years

1. Renal parenchymal diseases
2. Renovascular disease
3. Essential hypertension
4. Coarctation of the aorta
5. Endocrine causes
6. Iatrogenic (e.g. medications, postoperative hypertension).

### 14.33.5. Causes of hypertension 12–18 years

1. Essential hypertension
2. Iatrogenic
3. Renal parenchymal diseases
4. Renovascular disease
5. Endocrine causes
6. Coarctation of the aorta.

## 14.34. Causes of Renal Hypertension

Causes of renal hypertension

1. Chronic renal failure and postrenal transplant
2. Renal parenchymal disease
    a. Scarring due to reflux nephropathy or obstructive uropathy
    b. Acute or chronic glomerulonephritis
    c. Hemolytic uremic syndrome
    d. Renal dysplasia
    e. Polycystic kidneys.
3. Renovascular disease
    a. Renal artery stenosis
    b. Renal artery thrombosis
    c. Renal artery aneurysm
    d. Arteriovenous fistula.
4. Renal tumors
    a. Nephroblastoma
    b. Hamartoma
    c. Hemangiopericytoma.

## 14.35. Biochemical Urine Indices in Renal Failure

|  | Prerenal | Renal |
|---|---|---|
| Urine osmolality (mOsm/kg) | > 500 | < 350 |
| Urine Na (mmol/L) | < 20 | > 40 |
| U/P creatinine | > 40 | < 20 |
| U/P urea | > 15 | < 5 |
| $\mathrm{FeNa}^{+} = \dfrac{\mathrm{UNa} \times \mathrm{PCr}}{\mathrm{PNa} \times \mathrm{UCr}}$ | < 1% | > 3% |

## 14.36. Guidelines on the Indications for Dialysis

1. Uncontrollable fluid overload/hypertension.
2. Uncontrollable acidosis.
3. Symptomatic electrolyte disturbances not controlled by above measures.
4. Symptomatic uremia.
5. Presence of a dialyzable toxin.
6. Established anuria, even if 1–5 not present, provided obstruction excluded.

## 14.37. Stages of Chronic Renal Failure (CRF)

| Stage of CRF | GFR (mL/min/1.73 m$^2$) | Features |
|---|---|---|
| Mild | 50–75 | Asymptomatic |
| Moderate | 25–50 | Metabolic abnormalities |
| Severe | < 25 | Progressive growth failure |
| End-stage renal failure | < 10 | Require renal replacement therapy |

## Bibliography


1. http://kidney.niddk.nih.gov/kudiseases/pubs/biopsy/
2. http://www.deflux.com/country/usa/?q=node/50
3. http://www.edrep.org/pages/textbook/anaemia.php
4. http://www.emedicinehealth.com/cystoscopy/article_em.htm
5. http://www.kidney.niddk.nih.gov/kudiseases/pubs/tubularacidosis/
6. http://www.radiologyinfo.org/en/info.cfm?pg=voidcysto

## 15.1.  MRI of the Head

1.  May detect cerebral dysgenesis at any age in a child
2.  Consider it if any of the following are  present
* Cerebral palsy
* Abnormal head shape or size
* Craniofacial malformation
* Seizures
* Loss or stagnation of  developmental skills
* Neurocutaneous abnormalities
* IQ < 50.

## 15.2.  Cytogenetic Chromosome Testing for Mental Retardation

If mental retardation is present, do cytogenetic chromosome testing if any of the following is also found:
* Microcephaly
* Family history of mental retardation
* Family history of fetal loss
* IQ <50
* Skin pigmentary abnormalities
* Suspected genetic syndrome.

## 15.3.  Delayed Language Development

* 50% of children with delayed language development will have delays in other areas.
* Common causes of language development problems:
    – Hearing deficiency (always order the hearing first)
    – Mental retardation
    – Dysphasia
    – Dysarthria
    – Structural problems of the mouth/respiratory tract
    – Child abuse/neglect.

## 15.4.  Diagnostic Criteria for Migraine Headaches

Two of the following criteria are mandatory to diagnose migraine headaches.

- Pain on one side (although children with migraine can have bifrontal or bitemporal pain).
- Pulsating/throbbing character.
- Moderate-to-severe intensity.
- Increasing severity with activity.

## 15.5.  Febrile Infection-related Epilepsy Syndrome (FIRES)

The clinical characteristic best conceptualized FIRES as a chronic epilepsy with an explosive onset include:

- The similar perirolandic and perisylvian features of acute and chronic seizures.
- The lack of a silent period.
- The absence of evidence of cerebral inflammation.
- The poor response to immunotherapies.

## 15.6.  EEG Series

### 15.6.1.  Absence seizure

Note the asymmetrical left frontal onset.

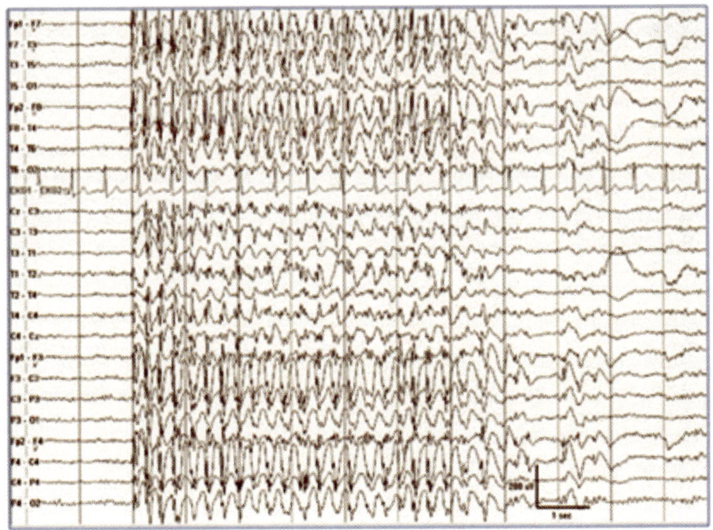

**Fig. 15.1**: EEG graph of absence seizure

### 15.6.1.1. Absence (Petit mal) seizure in an 8-year-old boy

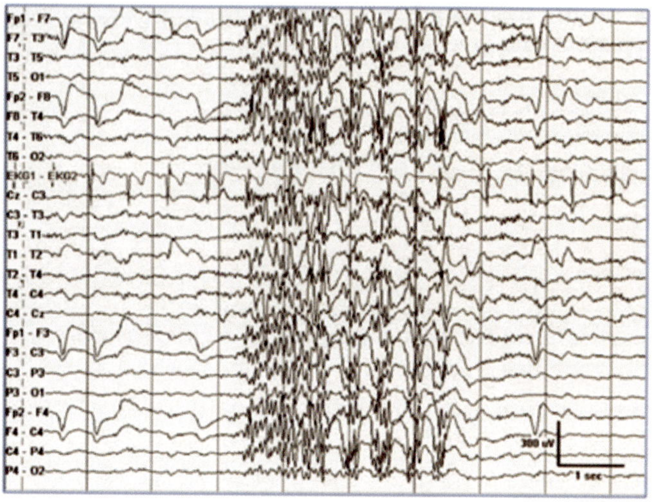

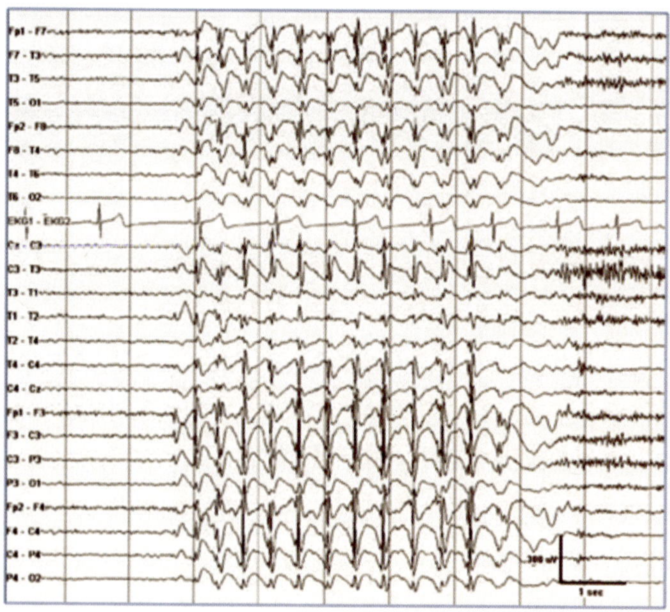

Fig. 15.2: EEG of absence seizure in an 8 year old boy

### 15.6.1.2. Atypical absence seizure in a patient with encephalopathic generalized epilepsy

Notice the polyspikes that evolve to a slow spike-and-wave pattern.

Fig. 15.3: EEG of atypical absence seizure

## 15.6.2. Myoclonic seizure

Myoclonic seizure associated with a burst of generalized polyspike-and-waves in a patient with juvenile myoclonic epilepsy (JME).

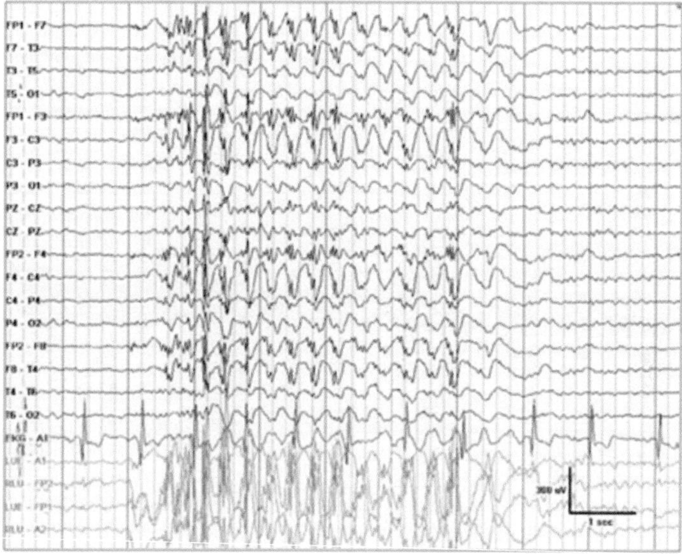

**Fig. 15.4**: EEG of myoclonic seizure

## 15.6.3. Infantile spasm

Infantile spasm noted in second 7 below with an electrodecremental response obtained in a 3-year-old child with tuberous sclerosis. Note the high amplitude.

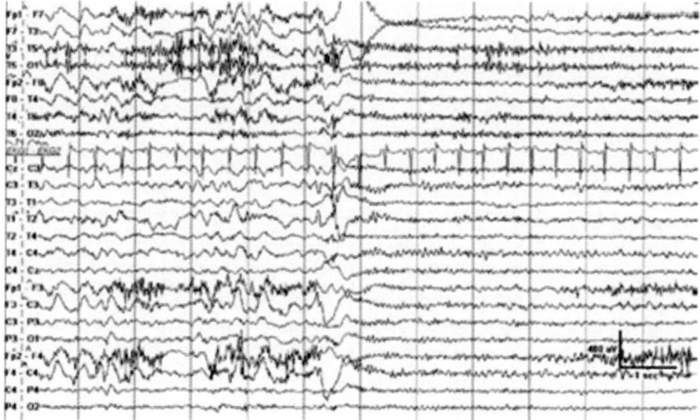

**Fig. 15.5**: EEG of infantile spasm

### 15.6.4. Lennox-Gastaut syndrome

Tonic seizure in a patient with Lennox-Gastaut syndrome.

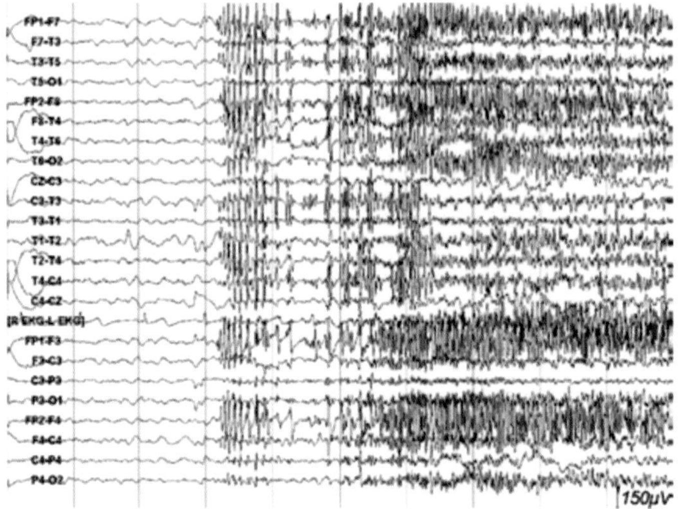

**Fig. 15.6**: EEG of Lennox-Gastaut syndrome

### 15.6.5. Simple partial seizure

The below EEG shows a simple partial seizure that occurred out of stage 2 sleep.

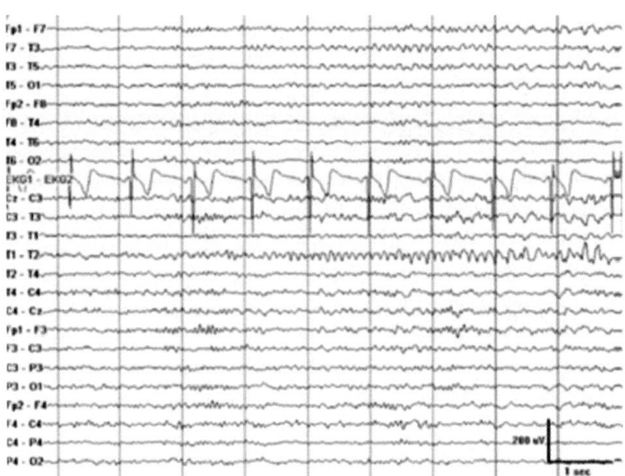

**Fig. 15.7**: EEG of simple partial seizure

## 15.6.6. Temporal lobe epilepsy

Right temporal 6- to 7-Hz rhythmic ictal theta discharge at seizure onset in a patient with temporal lobe epilepsy.

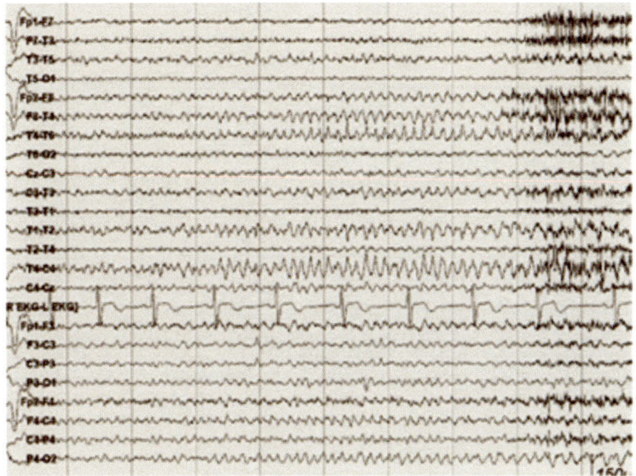

**Fig. 15.8**: EEG of temporal lobe epilepsy

## 15.6.7. Frontal lobe epilepsy

Nonlocalized ictal EEG in frontal lobe epilepsy.
Notice the brief right frontal-central repetitive spikes in seconds 7 to 8.

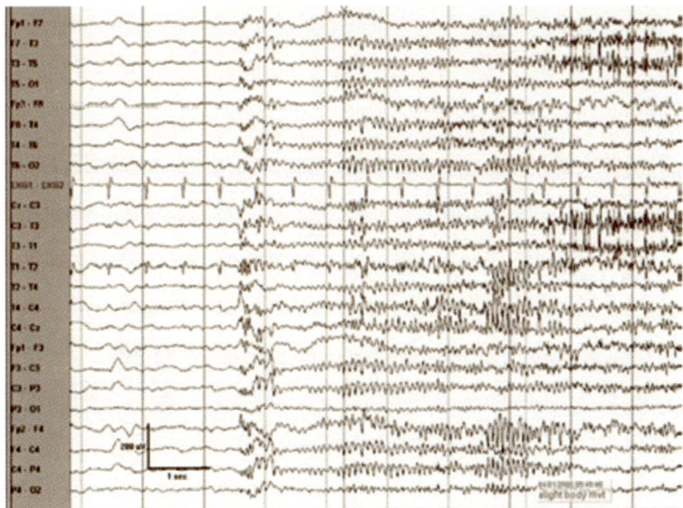

**Fig. 15.9**: EEG of frontal lobe epilepsy

## 15.7.    Screening Scheme for Developmental Delay: Upper Range

| Age (mo.) | Gross motor | Fine motor | Social skills | Language |
|---|---|---|---|---|
| 3 | Supports weight on forearms | Opens hands spontaneously | Smiles appropriately | Coos, laughs |
| 6 | Sits momentarily | Transfers objects | Shows likes and dislikes | Babbles |
| 9 | Pulls to stand | Pincer grasp | Plays pat-a-cake, peek-a-boo | Imitates sounds |
| 12 | Walks with one hand held | Releases an object on command | Comes when called | 1–2 meaningful words |
| 18 | Walks upstairs with assistance | Feeds from a spoon | Mimics actions of others | At least 6 words |
| 24 | Runs | Builds a tower of 6 blocks | Plays with others | 2–3-word sentences |

## 15.8.    Head Growth

### 15.8.1.  The average rate of head growth in a healthy premature infant

- 0.5 cm in the 1st 2 week.
- 0.75 cm in the 3rd week.
- 1.0 cm in the 4th week and every week thereafter until the 40th week of development.

### 15.8.2.  The head circumference of an average term infant

- Measures 34–35 cm at birth
- 44 cm at 6 month
- 47 cm at 1 year of age.

## 15.9.    Permanent Causes of Anosmia (Loss of Smell)

1. Head trauma with damage to the ethmoid bone or shearing of the olfactory nerve fibers as they cross the cribriform plate.
2. Tumors of the frontal lobe.
3. Intranasal drug use.
4. Exposure to toxins (acrylates, methacrylates and cadmium).

5. Occasionally, a child who recovers from purulent.
6. Meningitis or develops hydrocephalus has a diminished.
7. Sense of smell.
8. Rarely, anosmia is congenital (isolated deficit) or as part of Kallman syndrome (a familial disorder) characterized by:
    i. Hypogonadotropic hypogonadism
    ii. Congenital anosmia.

## 15.10. Horner Syndrome

### 15.10.1. Characterized by

1. Ipsilateral ptosis (droopy eyelid)
2. Miosis (constricted pupil)
3. Anhidrotic (lack of sweating) of the face.

### 15.10.2. Horner syndrome may be

1. Congenital
2. May be caused by a lesion of the sympathetic pathway in the:
    – Hypothalamus
    – Brainstem, cervical spinal cord
    – Sympathetic plexus.

## 15.11. Causes of True or Apparent VIth Nerve Weakness in Children

- VIth cranial nerve paresis:
    – Raised intracranial pressure
    – Brainstem glioma.
- Moebius syndrome
- Duane's syndrome
- Esotropia (abduction is usually normal).

## 15.12. Most Common Clinical Features of Progressive Infantile Hydrocephalus

### 15.12.1. 50% of progressive infantile hydrocephalus cases are asymptomatic

### 15.12.2. Symptoms of progressive infantile hydrocephalus

- Headache or irritability
- Vomiting

- Anorexia
- Drowsiness or lethargy.

### 15.12.3. Signs of progressive infantile hydrocephalus

- Inappropriately increasing occipitofrontal circumference (approx 75%).
- Tense anterior fontanelle.
- Splayed sutures.
- Scalp vein distension.
- Sunsetting (loss of upward gaze).
- Neck retraction or rigidity.
- Pupillary changes.
- Neurogenic stridor.
- Decerebration.

## 15.13.  Clinical Features of Decompensated Hydrocephalus (Children with Shunts)

### 15.13.1. Symptoms of decompensated hydrocephalus

- Vomiting
- Drowsiness or lethargy
- Headache
- Behavioral change
- Anorexia
- Valve malfunction
- Sleep disturbance
- Seizures.

### 15.13.2. Signs of decompensated hydrocephalus

- No clinical signs (approx 25%)
- Decreased conscious level
- Acute squint
- Neck retraction
- Distended retinal veins
- Sluggish palpable valve mechanism.

## 15.14.  Causes of Acquired Hydrocephalus

1. Posthemorrhagic causes
   - Neonatal intraventricular hemorrhage

- Subarachnoid hemorrhage
- Subdural hemorrhage.

2. Postmeningitic
   - Toxoplasmosis
   - Mumps (aqueductitis, ependymitis)
   - Pyogenic organisms (pneumococcus, haemophilus, etc.)
   - Cytomegalovirus
   - Other viral meningitides
   - Rubella
   - Tuberculous meningitis and tuberculoma.

3. Space-occupying lesions
   - Tumor
   - Clot
   - Cyst
   - Abscess.

4. Postasphyxial
   - Injury.

## 15.15.  Dandy-Walker Malformation

### 15.15.1. This incorporates

1. Cystic dilation of the fourth ventricle.
2. An enlarged posterior fossa with upward displacement of the tentorium.
3. Cerebellar vermian hypoplasia.

### 15.15.2. Facts on Dandy-Walker malformation

- A definitive diagnosis cannot be made until after 18 weeks' gestation as normal cerebellar hemisphere fusion is not complete until 17 weeks' gestation.
- There is an association of Dandy-Walker malformations with chromosomal abnormality in upto 45%.
- The outcome for Dandy-Walker malformations and its variants ranges from normal to severe disability.

## 15.16. Classification of Spina Bifida

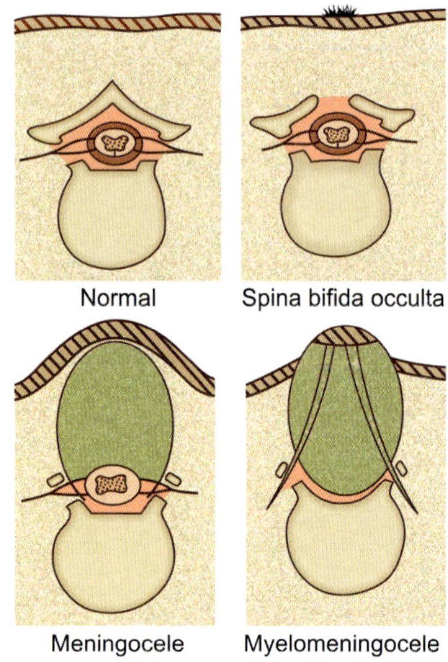



**Fig. 15.10**: Types of spina bifida

## 15.17. Neurofibromatosis 1 (NF1)

### 15.17.1. Incidence of NF1

NF1 is the most common single gene disorder to affect the human nervous system with an estimated incidence of 1 in 3000.

### 15.17.2. Genetics of NF1

- This is an autosomal dominant disorder although 50% of cases are sporadic.
- The NF1 gene has been mapped to chromosome 17 and codes the protein neurofibromin.

### 15.17.3. Diagnostic criteria for NF1: Two or more of the following are required

1. Six or more café-au-lait spots (at least 1.5 cm postpuberty, at least 0.5 cm prepuberty).
2. Two or more neurofibromas or one or more plexiform neurofibromata.
3. Axillary or inguinal freckling.
4. Optic glioma.

5. Two or more Lisch nodules (benign iris hamartomas).
6. Osseous dysplasia on the sphenoid bone or cortex of a long bone.
7. A first degree relative with NF1.

## 15.18. Neurofibromatosis 2 (NF2)

### 15.18.1. Incidence and genetics of NF2

- NF2 is very rare with a birth incidence of 1 in 40 000.
- It shows autosomal dominant transmission with nearly full pene-trance.
- The NF2 gene maps to the long arm of chromosome 22 and codes a member of the protein 4.1 family of cytoskeletal associated elements.

### 15.18.2. The diagnosis for NF2 is based on the following criteria

1. Bilateral VIIIth nerve masses detected on neuroimaging.
2. A first degree relative with NF2 and either unilateral VIIIth nerve mass or two of the following:
   i. Neurofibroma
   ii. Meningioma
   iii. Glioma
   iv. Schwannoma
   v. Juvenile posterior subcapsular lenticular opacity.

## 15.19. Diagnostic Criteria for Tuberous Sclerosis Complex (TSC)

### 15.19.1. Major features

1. Facial or forehead plaque
2. Nontraumatic ungual or periungual fibroma
3. Hypomelanotic macules (more than three)
4. Shagreen patch (connective tissue nevus)
5. Multiple retinal nodular hamartoma
6. Cortical tuber
7. Subependymal nodule
8. Subependymal giant cell astrocytoma
9. Cardiac rhabdomyoma, single or multiple
10. Lymphangiomyomatosis
11. Renal angiomyolipoma.

### 15.19.2. Minor features

1. Multiple randomly distributed pits in dental enamel
2. Hamartomatous rectal polyps
3. Bone cyst

4. Cerebral white matter radial migration lines
5. Gingival fibromas
6. Nonrenal hamartoma
7. Retinal achromic patches
8. 'Confetti' skin lesions
9. Multiple renal cysts.

### 15.19.3. Criteria for diagnosis of tuberous sclerosis complex (TSC)

- Definite TCS—Either two major features or one major feature plus two minor features.
- Probable TCS—One major plus one minor feature.
- Possible TCS—Either one major feature or two minor features.

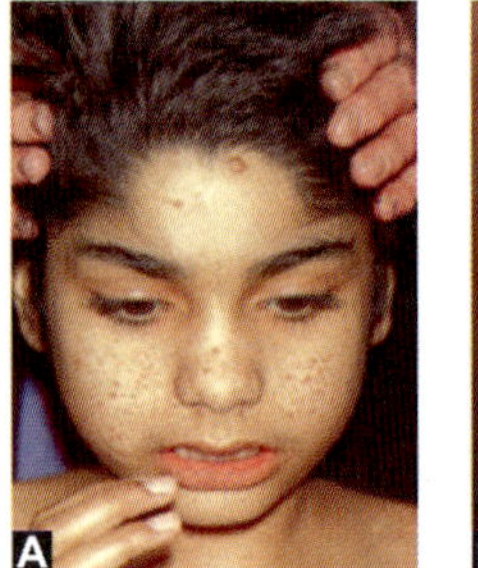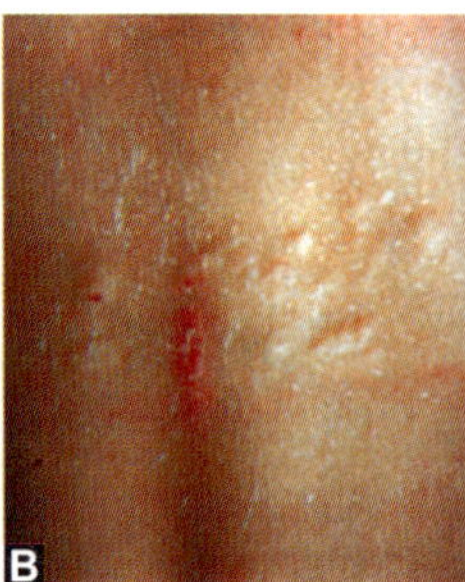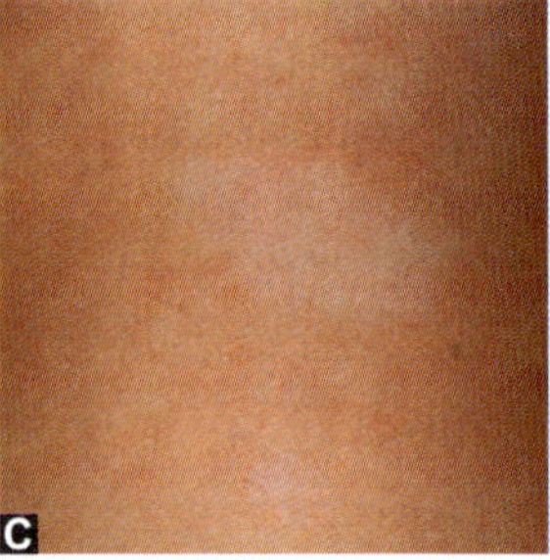

**Figs 15.11A to C**: Tuberous sclerosis—Various skin lesions

## 15.20. Principal Purposes for the Usage of EEG, to

- Help establish the likely diagnosis of epilepsy
- Help establish the type of epilepsy
- Help identify possible precipitants to epileptic seizures
- Investigate the cause of cognitive decline
- Help localize the onset of focal seizures
- Monitor treatment, including the timing of drug withdrawal.

## 15.21. Generalized, Self-limited Seizures

### 15.21.1. Generalized tonic-clonic seizures (GTCS)

- Involve an initial, bilaterally symmetrical, sustained contraction of the muscles (tonic phase) followed by bilateral repetitive, rhythmical contractions of the limbs (clonic phase).

- There is usually a phase of postictal drowsiness, of variable duration.
- During GTCS, manifestations such as tongue biting, cyanosis of the lips and incontinence are frequent.

## 15.21.2. Tonic seizures

- Characterized by sustained muscle contractions lasting a few seconds to minutes.
- It may involve the whole, or greater part, of the body or be confined to particular parts of the body.
- Tonic seizures may be manifested by opisthotonus or by a subtle elevation of the eyebrows.

## 15.21.3. Clonic seizures

- Manifested by rhythmical contractions of the limbs
- An alternative term is rhythmic myoclonus.

## 15.21.4. Myoclonic seizures

- Characterized by sudden, brief (<100 ms), involuntary, single or multiple contraction(s) of muscle(s) or muscle groups.
- They may be massive, involving axial and proximal limb muscles, or subtle and fragmentary involving distal muscles.

### Special types of myoclonic seizure

#### *15.21.4.1.  Myoclonic absence seizures*

Characterized by a typical absence seizure with rhythmical myoclonus usually involving the head and proximal muscle of the upper limbs.

#### *15.21.4.2.  Eyelid myoclonia*

Characterized by rhythmical myoclonia of the eyelids sometimes accompanied by a brief typical absence seizure.

#### *15.21.4.3.  Myoclonic atonic seizures*

Consisting of a brief jerk followed by a diffuse loss of tone.

## 15.21.5. Atonic seizures

Characterized by a sudden diminution of muscle tone lasting a second or longer, and involving the head, trunk, jaw or limb musculature.

### 15.21.6. Epileptic spasms (previously called infantile spasms)

- Consist of a sudden flexion, extension or mixed extension-flexion of, predominantly proximal and truncal, muscles which is more sustained than myoclonus but briefer than a tonic seizure (approx 1s).
- They frequently occur in clusters and it is now recognized that their occurrence is not limited to infancy or to West syndrome.

### 15.21.7. Absence seizures

- Characterized clinically by a brief impairment of consciousness.
- The depth of impairment of consciousness during absences varies.
- Unless mild, automatisms are frequent.
- Mild clonic, myoclonic, and atonic phenomena may also occur during absences.

*Automatisms (defined as more or less coordinated, repetitive, motor activity usually occurring when cognition is impaired and for which the subject is usually amnesic afterwards.*

- They are usually relatively simple, e.g. lip smacking and fumbling with hands.

### 15.21.7.1. Typical absence seizures

- Brief impairment of consciousness is of abrupt onset and cessation with no postictal symptoms.
- Typical absence seizures are accompanied, on the EEG, by generalized 3-Hz spike-wave discharges.

### 15.21.7.2. Atypical absence seizures

- Onset and cessation of the brief impairment of consciousness may be less clearly defined, with the person appearing to drift into and out of the seizure.
- Atypical absence seizures are usually accompanied by generalized spike-wave discharges at frequencies under 2.5 Hz.

## 15.22.  Focal, Self-limited Seizures

### 15.22.1. Focal motor seizures

- Involve muscle activity in any form, with either an increase or decrease in muscle contraction.

## FOCAL MOTOR SEIZURES SUBTYPES INCLUDE

### *15.22.1.1. Focal motor seizures with elementary clonic motor signs*

- Imply involvement of the primary motor area of the frontal lobe and may include a Jacksonian march with spread of clonic movements through contiguous body parts.

*'Elementary' implies that a single type of contraction of a muscle or group of muscles is involved 'Clonic' implies regular repetitive contractions.*

### *15.22.1.2. Focal motor seizures with asymmetrical tonic motor signs*

- Characterized by an asymmetrical, sustained increase in muscle contractions, causing, e.g. the child to adopt a 'fencing' posture.
- They are characteristic of those involving the supplementary motor areas of the frontal lobes although they can arise from other frontal lobe regions and from extrafrontal lobe sites.

### *15.22.1.3. Focal motor seizures with typical (temporal lobe) automatisms*

- Occurs in mesial temporal lobe seizures.

### *15.22.1.4. Focal motor seizures with hyperkinetic automatisms*

- Such seizures usually imply a frontal lobe origin
- Such as pedalling, thrashing and rocking movements.

### *15.22.1.5. Rarer seizure types*

- Focal negative myoclonus.
- Seizures with inhibitory motor signs (implying a loss of muscle contraction as in motor arrest).

### 15.22.2. Focal sensory seizures

- Characterized by a perceptual experience not caused by appropriate stimuli in the external world.

## FOCAL SENSORY SEIZURES SUBTYPE INCLUDE

### *15.22.2.1. Focal sensory seizures with elementary sensory symptoms*

Here the term 'elementary' is used to imply a single, unformed pheno-menon involving one primary sensory modality, e.g. somatosensory (parietal lobe seizures), visual (occipital lobe seizures), auditory, olfactory, gustatory, epigastric or cephalic.

### *15.22.2.2. Focal motor seizures with experiential sensory symptoms*

- These are characteristic of seizures involving the junction of the temporal, parietal and occipital lobes.e.g.:
    - i. Affective symptoms (fear, depression, anger, etc.).
    - ii. Distortions of reality (déjà vu, jamais vu).
    - iii. Feelings of depersonalization and formed illusionary or hallucinatory events.

### 15.22.3. Gelastic seizures

- Characterized by ictal laughter or giggling, usually without an appropriate affective tone.
- Such seizures often involve the hypothalamus.

### 15.22.4. Hemiclonic seizures

- Characterized by rhythmical clonic jerking involving one side of the body.

### 15.22.5. Secondary, generalized seizures

- Seizures whose onset is focal (e.g. motor or sensory) and then becomes generalized, usually as a tonic-clonic seizure.

### 15.22.6. Autonomic seizures

- Characterized by altered autonomic function (objective or subjective) of any type (cardiovascular, pupillary, gastrointestinal, sudomotor, vasomotor and thermoregularity) at seizure onset or in which all manifestations are consistent with altered autonomic function.

## 15.23.  Indications for Neuroimaging in Children with Headache

Indications for neuroimaging in children with headache
1. Features of cerebellar dysfuction: ataxia; nystagmus; intention tremor.
2. Features of increased intracranial pressure: papilledema; night or early morning vomiting; large head.
3. New focal or new neurological deficits including recent squint.
4. Seizures and specially focal.
5. Personality change.
6. Deterioration of school work.

## 15.24.  Causes of Ataxia in Children

### 15.24.1. Metabolic causes of ataxia in children

1.  Any cause of fat malabsorption
2.  Neuronal ceroid lipofuscinosis (late infantile)
3.  Abetalipoproteinemia
4.  Vitamin E deficiency
5.  Biotinidase deficiency
6.  Mitochondrial cytopathies
7.  Metachromatic leukodystrophy
8.  Refsum disease
9.  Organic acidemias
10.  Sialidosis
11.  Urea cycle disorders.

### 15.24.2. Acute/subacute causes of ataxia in children

1.  Acute cerebellar ataxia
2.  Acute labyrinthitis hydrocephalus
3.  Posterior fossa tumor/space occupying lesion
4.  Traumatic brain injury
5.  Acute disseminated encephalomyelitis
6.  Toxic/poisoning
7.  Miller-Fisher syndrome
8.  Nonconvulsive status
9.  Postinfectious polyneuropathy
10.  Acute labyrinthitis.

## 15.25.  Transient Movement Disorders in Childhood

1.  Benign paroxysmal torticollis of infancy
2.  Benign myoclonus of the newborn
3.  Benign myoclonus of infancy
4.  Jitteriness
5.  Transient paroxysmal dystonia of infancy
6.  Spasmus nutans.

## Bibliography


1. http://www.emedicinehealth.com/migraine_headache/article_em.htm
2. http://www.medindia.net/patients/patientinfo/anosmia_causes.htm
3. http://www.medscape.com/viewarticle/504722
4. http://www.ncbi.nlm.nih.gov/pubmed/14679581
5. http://www.ncbi.nlm.nih.gov/pubmed/20345937
6. http://www.nidcd.nih.gov/health/voice/pages/speechandlanguage.aspx
7. www.foreverinmomgenes.com

## 16.1. Common Chemotherapeutic Agents; Mechanism of Action and Toxicity

| Drug | Mechanism of action | Toxicity |
|---|---|---|
| **Antimetabolites** | | |
| Methotrexate | Folic acid antagonist | Myelosuppression |
| 6-MP | Inhibits purine synthesis | |
| Ara-C | Inhibits DNA polymerase | |
| **Alkylating agents** | | |
| Cyclophosphamide | Inhibits DNA synthesis | Hemorrhagic cystitis |
| **Antibiotics** | | |
| Doxorubicin | Binds to DNA | Cardiomyopathy |
| Daunorubicin | | |
| Bleomycin | | Pulmonary fibrosis |
| **Vinca alkaloids** | | |
| Vincristine | Inhibits microtubule formation | Peripheral neuropathy |
| Vinblastine | | Leukopenia |
| **Enzymes** | | |
| L-asparaginase | Depletes L-asparagine | Pancreatitis, increased glucose |
| **Hormones** | | |
| Prednisone | Unknown | 1. Cushing syndrome<br>2. Cataracts<br>3. Diabetes mellitus (DM)<br>4. Hypertension (HTN) |
| **Other** | | |
| Cisplatin | Inhibits DNA synthesis | {NON}<br>1. Nephrotoxic<br>2. Ototoxic<br>3. Neurotoxic |
| Etoposide (VP-16) | Topoisomerase inhibitor | Secondary leukemias |

## 16.2.  Some Conditions Predispose to AML

- Trisomy 21
- Diamond-Blackfan syndrome
- Fanconi anemia
- Bloom syndrome
- Kostmann syndrome
- Paroxysmal nocturnal hemoglobinuria
- Neurofibromatosis.

## 16.3.  Differences between Osteosarcoma and Ewing Sarcoma

|  | Osteosarcoma | Ewing sarcoma |
|---|---|---|
| Race | All races | Caucasians |
| Age | Children and adolescents | Less than 10 years |
| Cell type | Spindle cell-producing osteoid | Undifferentiated, probably neural |
| Site | Metaphyses of long bones | Diaphyses of long and flat bones |
| Presentation | 1. History of injury<br>2. Local pain/swelling | 1. Fever<br>2. Local pain/swelling |
| X-ray findings | Less commonly lytic, "Sunburst" pattern | Lytic "Onion skinning" |

## 16.4.  The Most Common Signs and Symptoms of Cancer in Children

- Pallor, bruising, persistent fever or infection; pancytopenia.
- Pain: Persistent and unexplained; metastasis, bone marrow malignancy and primary bone tumor.
- Headache with neurologic deficit.
- Morning headache and vomiting; increased intracranial pressure.
- Lymphadenopathy: Persistent and unexplained.
- Abdominal mass.
- Mass or persistent swelling.
- Eye changes: Proptosis and white papillary reflex.

## 16.5. Uncommon Signs and Symptoms of Cancer in Children

### 16.5.1. Uncommon signs and symptoms of cancer in children related directly to tumor

- Superior vena cava syndrome
- Subcutaneous nodules
- Leukemoid reaction
- Myasthenia gravis
- Heterochromia.

### 16.5.2. Uncommon signs and symptoms of cancer in children not related directly to tumor

- Chronic diarrhea
- Polymyoclonus-opsoclonus
- Failure to thrive
- Cushing syndrome
- Pseudomuscular dystrophy.

## 16.6. Oncologic Emergencies

### 16.6.1. Metabolic

- Hyperuricemia
- Hyperkalemia
- Hyperphosphatemia
- Hyponatremia
- Hypercalcemia.

### 16.6.2. Hematologic

- Anemia
- Thrombocytopenia
- Disseminated intravascular coagulation
- Neutropenia
- Hyperleukocytosis ($> 50,000/mm^3$)
- Graft versus host disease.

### 16.6.3. Space-occupying lesions

- Spinal cord compression
- Increased intracranial pressure

- Superior vena cava syndrome
- Tracheal compression.

## 16.7. Potential Long-term Sequelae of Childhood Cancer

1. Late recurrence of primary cancer.
2. Second malignancy.
3. Impairment of normal growth.
4. Endocrine dysfunction.
5. Infertility.
6. Educational and psychological dysfunction.
7. Other organ toxicity, e.g. cardiac, pulmonary.
8. Impairment of normal life, e.g. obtaining work, insurance, being allowed to adopt children.

## 16.8.   Categorical  Etiological Factors for CNS Tumors

### 16.8.1.  Heritable syndromes as etiological factors for CNS tumors

1. Neurofibromatosis (visual pathway tumors + gliomas)
2. Tuberous sclerosis (glial ependymomas)
3. Von Hippel-Lindau (cerebellar + retinal + pheochromocytomas).

### 16.8.2.  Immunodeficiency (intracerebral lymphomas) as etiological factors for CNS tumors specially

a. Postrenal transplantation
b. Wiskott-Aldrich
c. Ataxia telangiectasia.

## 16.9.   The WHO Classification Hodgkin's Lymphoma or Hodgkin's Disease (HD)

**According to the WHO classification HD can be subdivided into four subtypes**

1. Lymphocyte predominance:
    i. Reed-Sternberg cells may be quite scarce
    ii. Fibrosis is rarely seen
    iii. The prognosis is very good.
2. Mixed cellularity:
    i. Reed-Sternberg cells are usually profuse (5–15 per high power field).
    ii. Often with fine fibrosis and focal necrosis.

3.  Lymphocyte depletion:
    i.   Large abnormal mononuclear cells are often seen as well as Reed-Sternberg cells with few lymphocytes.
    ii.  Fibrosis and necrosis are common and often quite diffuse.
    iii. This form is rarer in children.
4.  Nodular sclerosis:
    i.   Lacunar cells are a characteristic finding with a thickened capsule and bands which divide the tissue into nodules.
    ii.  This histology is specially common in lower cervical, supra-clavicular and mediastinal HD of childhood.

## 16.10. Factors  Predisposing to Childhood Leukemia

### 16.10.1.  Genetic conditions predisposing to childhood leukemia

| | |
|---|---|
| Down syndrome | Neurofibromatosis type I |
| Fanconi anemia | Ataxia-telangiectasia |
| Bloom syndrome | Severe combined immune deficiency |
| Diamond-Blackfan anemia | Paroxysmal nocturnal hemoglobinuria |
| Schwachman-Diamond syndrome | Li-Fraumeni syndrome |
| Kostmann syndrome | |

### 16.10.2.  Environmental conditions predisposing to childhood leukemia

| | |
|---|---|
| Ionizing radiation | Nitrosourea |
| Drugs | Epipodophyllotoxin |
| Alkylating agents | Benzene exposure |
| Advanced maternal age (?) | |

## 16.11. French-American-British (FAB) Classification of Acute Myelogenous Leukemia

| Subtype | Common name |
|---|---|
| M0 | Acute myeloblastic leukemia without differentiation |
| M1 | Acute myeloblastic leukemia without maturation |
| M2 | Acute myeloblastic leukemia with maturation |

*Contd...*

*Contd...*

| Subtype | Common name |
|---------|-------------|
| M3 | Acute promyeloblastic leukemia |
| M4 | Acute myelomonocytic leukemia |
| M5 | Acute monocytic leukemia |
| M6 | Erythroleukemia |
| M7 | Acute megakaryocytic leukemia |

## 16.12. Location of Childhood Brain Tumors within the Central Nervous System

The relative frequency of brain tumor histologic types and the anatomic distribution are shown:

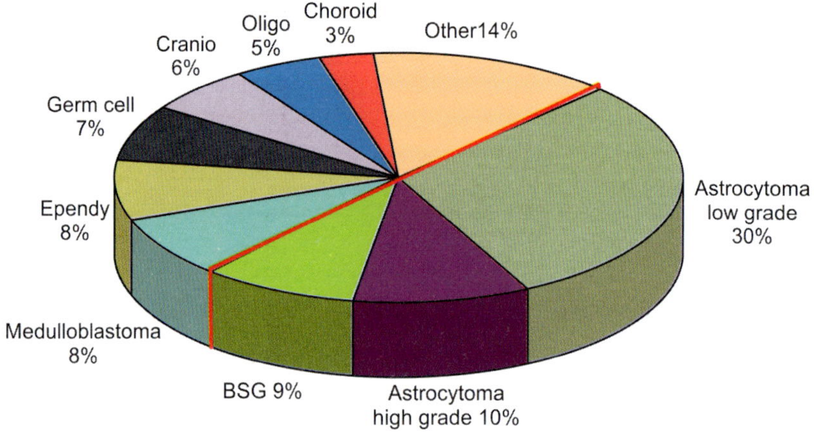


**Fig. 16.1**: The relative frequency of brain tumor histologic types and the anatomic distribution

## Bibliography


1. https://www.caring4cancer.com/go/cancer/treatment/chemotherapy/common-chemotherapy-drugs-and-side-effects.htm
2. http://www.medscape.com/viewarticle/453273
3. http://www.ncbi.nlm.nih.gov/books/NBK20928/
4. http://www.ncbi.nlm.nih.gov/pmc/articles/PMC1817663/
5. http://www.ncbi.nlm.nih.gov/pmc/articles/PMC474028/
6. http://www.scielo.br/scielo.php?script=sci_arttext&pid=S1807-59322006000200003
7. http://erc.endocrinology-journals.org/content/17/3/R141.full

# 17
# Ophthalmology

## 17.1. Useful Screening Questions for Older Children with Perceptual Visual Difficulties Related to Central Nervous System (CNS) Disease

**Does the child have difficulty:**

1. Identifying objects within a 'busy' or 'fast-moving' environment?
2. With coordination and movement in three-dimensional space?
3. Recognizing familiar faces?
4. With orientation in familiar environments?

## 17.2. Refractive Errors

### 17.2.1. Hypermetropia in infants

Most infants are slightly hypermetropic, which normally resolves by age 2 years—'emmetropization'.

### 17.2.2. Hypermetropia

Hypermetropia present after the age of 2 years normally persists into adult life.

### 17.2.3. Myopia is rare in young children

#### 17.2.3.1. *When high degrees of myopia do occur an underlying disease such as*

1. Homocystinuria
2. Marfan syndrome
3. Stickler syndrome
   should be considered.

### 17.2.4. Syndromes associated with hypermetropia or myopia

- Leber's congenital amaurosis is often associated with hypermetropia
- Marfan syndrome with myopia.

### 17.2.5. Signs and symptoms of refractive errors

- Blurred vision is the most common symptom of refractive errors
- Other symptoms may include the following:
    1. Double vision
    2. Haziness
    3. Glare or halos around bright lights
    4. Squinting
    5. Headaches
    6. Eye strain.

## 17.3.   Causes of Cerebral Visual Impairment

### 17.3.1. Prenatal

- Brain malformations
- Intrauterine infections
- Placental dysfunction.

### 17.3.2. Preterm neonatal

Preterm neonatal periventricular hemorrhage.

### 17.3.3. Perinatal

- Neonatal asphyxia
- Intracerebral hemorrhage
- Meningitis
- Encephalitis.

### 17.3.4. Postnatal

- Trauma (accidental and nonaccidental)
- Cardiac arrest.

## 17.4.   Conditions that may Present with (Apparent) Concomitant Strabismus

- Retinoblastoma
- Optic nerve hypoplasia
- Optic atrophy:
    - Primary
    - Secondary to neoplasm.

- Unilateral cataract
- Persistent fetal vasculature
- VIth cranial nerve weakness.

## 17.5.  Causes of True or Apparent VIth Nerve Weakness in Children

1. VIth cranial nerve paresis:
    i. Raised intracranial pressure
    ii. Brainstem glioma.
2. Moebius syndrome
3. Duane's syndrome
4. Esotropia (abduction is usually normal).

## 17.6.  Mnemonic 'DWARF' for Evaluation of Nystagmus

Nystagmus may be described using the mnemonic **'DWARF'**:

**D**irection (horizontal or vertical)

**W**ave form (jerk or pendular)

**A**mplitude (large amplitude or small amplitude oscillations)

**R**est (primary position (at rest/gaze evoked))

**F**requency (rapid movements or slow movements).

## 17.7.  Causes of Sensory Congenital Nystagmus

- Albinism
- Leber's amaurosis
- Aniridia
- Optic nerve hypoplasia
- Retinal cone dystrophy.

### 17.7.1. Albinism

Albinism refers to a group of conditions that may be divided into:
1. Oculocutaneous albinism (OCA)
2. Ocular albinism (OA).

**The ocular abnormalities found are common to all forms of albinism**
The ocular abnormalities include:
1. Defective iris and fundus pigmentation
2. Reduced vision and photophobia
3. Nystagmus
4. Strabismus
5. Delayed visual maturation

6. Foveal hypoplasia
7. Abnormal chiasmal crossing.

**Most forms of OCA are autosomal recessive**

Two rare forms of OCA are associated with systemic disease:

1. Chédiak-Higashi disease (increased susceptibility to infection).
2. Hermansky-Pudlak syndrome (frequent bruising due to platelet dysfunction).

## 17.8.  Causes of Acquired Nystagmus in Children

- Suprasellar tumor
- Posterior fossa tumor or malformation
- Neurodegenerative diseases such as:
    1. Batten's disease
    2. Neuroliposes
    3. Peroxisomal disorders.

## 17.9.  Ocular Defects that may Cause Bilateral Congenital Blindness

### 17.9.1. Whole globe

1. Anophthalmos
2. Microphthalmos.

### 17.9.2. Cornea

1. Sclerocornea
2. Peter's anomaly.

### 17.9.3. Lens

Cataract.

### 17.9.4. Retina

1. Retinal detachment (e.g. following retinopathy of prematurity)
2. Retinal dysplasia (e.g. Norrie's disease)
3. Chorioretinal coloboma
4. Chorioretinitis scarring
5. Cherry red spot in storage diseases (e.g. Tay-Sachs disease).

### 17.9.5. Optic atrophy

Prenatal:
1. Infection
2. Asphyxia
3. Cerebral malformations.

Perinatal:
1. Asphyxia.

Postnatal:
1. Meningitis/encephalitis
2. Compression (e.g. hydrocephalus and craniopharyngioma)
3. Genetic (e.g. autosomal dominant optic atrophy)
4. Secondry to retinal disease.

### 17.9.6. Optic nerve hypoplasia

Optic nerve hypoplasia is associated with maternal diabetes, maternal alcohol and drug abuse, maternal use of antiepileptic drugs, and young maternal age (20 years of age or less), most cases of ONH have no clearly identifiable cause.

### 17.9.7. Optic disk colobomas

The following conditions have been associated with optic disk coloboma:
1. Basal encephalocele.
2. Aicardi's syndrome.
3. CHARGE association (coloboma, heart defects, atresia choanae, retarded growth and development, genital hypoplasia, ear anomaly and deafness).
4. Goltz's focal dermal hypoplasia.
5. Meckel's syndrome.
6. Warburg's syndrome.
   Chromosome abnormalities such as trisomy 13 or 4p.

### 17.10. The Blind Infant with Apparently Normal Eyes

- Delayed visual maturation
- Cerebral visual impairment
- Leber's congenital amaurosis
- Retinal cone dystrophy
- Optic nerve hypoplasia
- Oculomotor praxia.

## 17.11. Causes of Visual Loss in Children Evident on Ophthalmic Examination

### 17.11.1. Cataract

Metabolic disease.

### 17.11.2. Retina

Retinal dystrophies
1. Rod-cone dystrophies
2. X-linked juvenile retinoschisis
3. Stargardt's disease.

### 17.11.3. Optic atrophy

1. External compression:
   Hydrocephalus tumor:
       Craniopharyngioma other suprasellar tumors.
2. Intrinsic tumor:
   Glioma:
       Neurofibromatosis type I.
3. Retinal diseases
4. Genetic
   Autosomal dominant optic atrophy.
5. Demyelinating diseases.

## 17.12. Congenital Ptosis

| Classification  of congenital ptosis | |
| --- | --- |
| 1.  Aponeurotic | Disinsertion of aponeurosis |
| 2.  Myogenic | • Localized dystrophy (most common)<br>• Other muscle diseases (myotonic dystrophy) |
| 3.  Neurogenic | • 3rd nerve palsy<br>• Horner's syndrome<br>• Jaw-wink ptosis |
| 4.  Neuromyogenic | Myasthenia gravis |
| 5.  Mechanical | Lid tumors |
| 6.  Pseudoptosis | • Microphthalmic eye, anophthalmos, phthisis bulbi<br>• Hypotropia<br>• Contralateral lid retraction<br>• Contralateral proptosis |

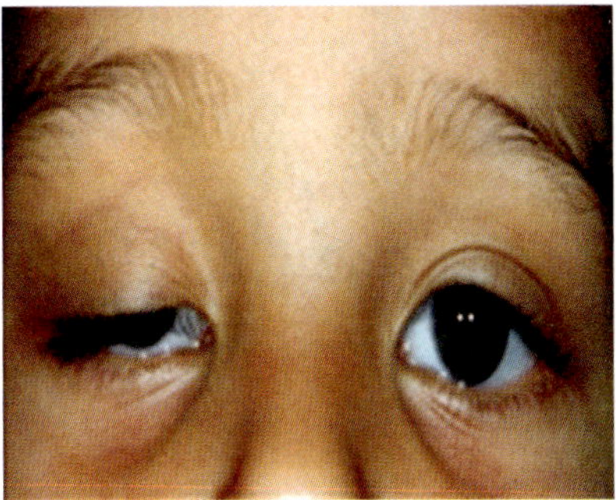

**Fig. 17.1**: Congenital ptosis

## 17.13. Causes of Congenital Cataracts

### 17.13.1. Inherited syndrome that cause congenital cataracts

- Chromosomal:
  - Trisomy 21,13,18
  - Turner's
  - Translocation 3;4 and 2;14
  - Cri du chat 5q15.2.
- Mitochondrial diseases
- Lowe's oculocerebrorenal syndrome
- Ectodermal dysplasia.

### 17.13.2. Metabolic diseases that cause congenital cataracts

- Galactosemia
- Galactokinase deficiency
- Hypocalcemia
- Hypoglycemia
- Mannosidosis.

### 17.13.3. Prenatal infection that cause congenital cataracts

- Rubella
- Toxoplasma
- Herpes simplex
- Varicella.

### 17.13.4. Trauma that cause congenital cataracts

- Accidental
- Nonaccidental

- Ocular associations
- Microphthalmos
- Aniridia
- Persistent fetal vasculature
- Peter's anomaly
- Endophthalmitis.

## 17.14. Abnormalities of the Optic Disk and Retina

### 17.14.1. Hypoplastic disk and optic nerve hypoplasia

The optic disk is anatomically very small in this case, with severely reduced vision.

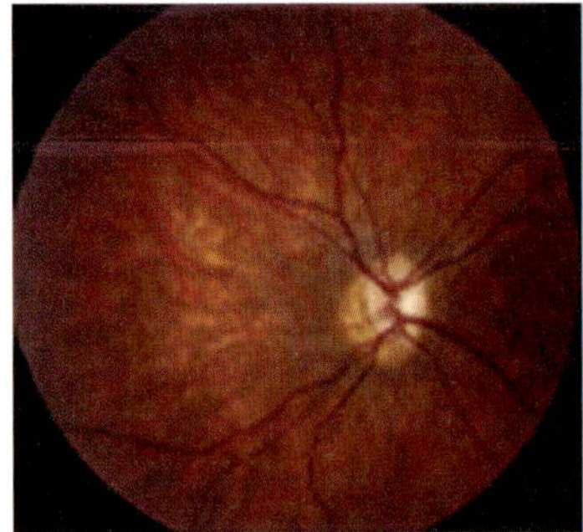

**Fig. 17.2**: Hypoplastic disk

### 17.14.2. Retinitis pigmentosa

Typical 'bone spicule' pigmentation is seen in the midperiphery of the fundus.

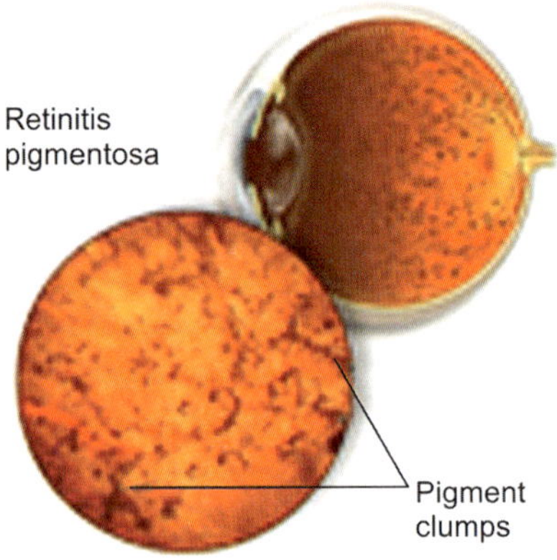


**Fig. 17.3**: Retinitis pigmentosa

### 17.14.3. Retinal cone dystrophy

With typical 'bull's eye' pigmentation at the center of the macula.

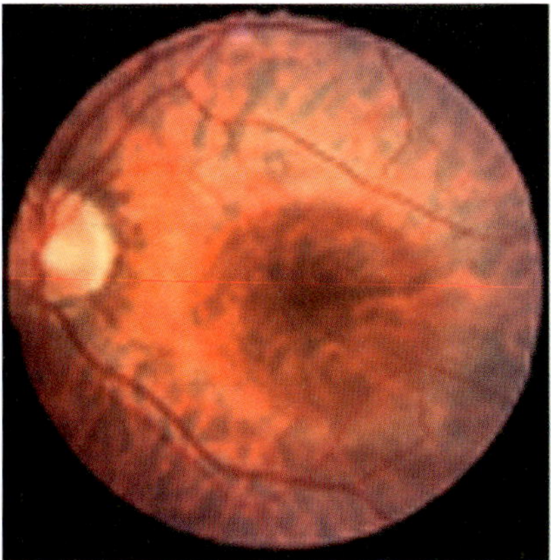

**Fig. 17.4**: Retinal cone dystrophy

### 17.14.4. Severe papilledema with hemorrhages and exudates

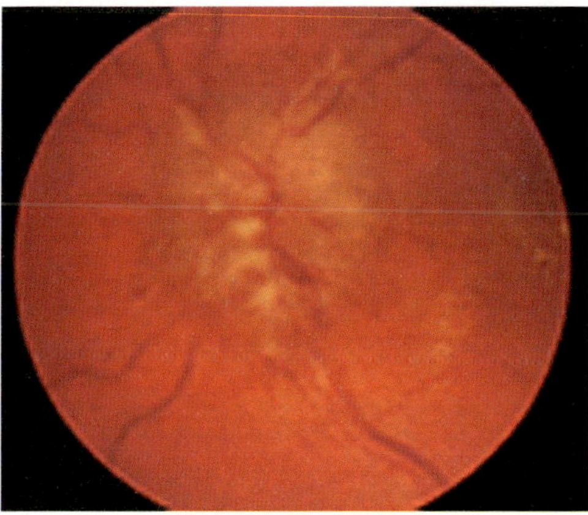

**Fig. 17.5**: Severe papilledema

### 17.14.5. Optic disk drusen

Optic nerve drusen are abnormal globular collections of protein and calcium salts which accumulate in the optic nerve and usually become visible after the first decade of life. They occur in both eyes more often than just one.

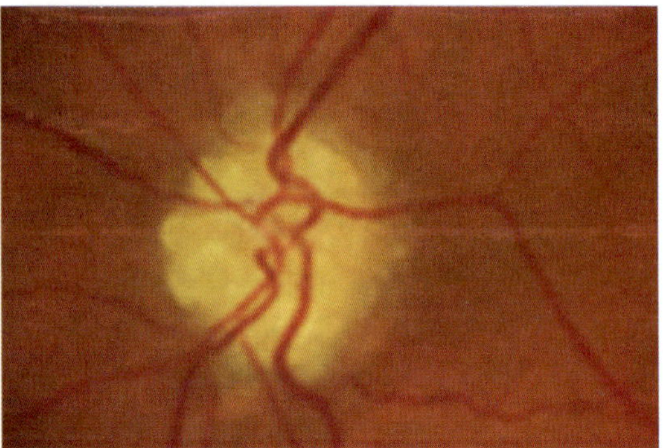

**Fig. 17.6**: Optic disk drusen

## 17.14.6. Cherry red spot due to Tay-Sachs disease

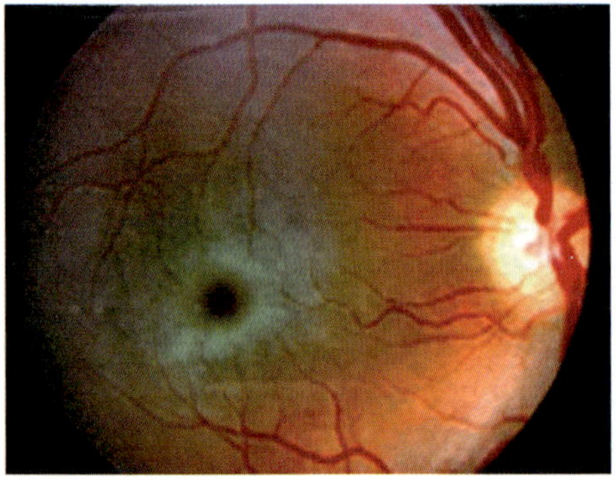

**Fig. 17.7**: Cherry red spot

## 17 .14.7. Retinal hemorrhages related to leukemia

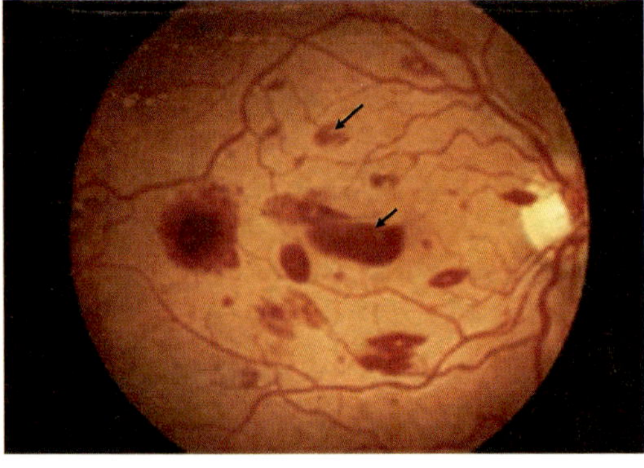

**Fig. 17.8**: Retinal hemorrhages

## 17.14.8. Large multinodular retinal hamartoma  adjacent to optic disk in a case of tuberous  sclerosis

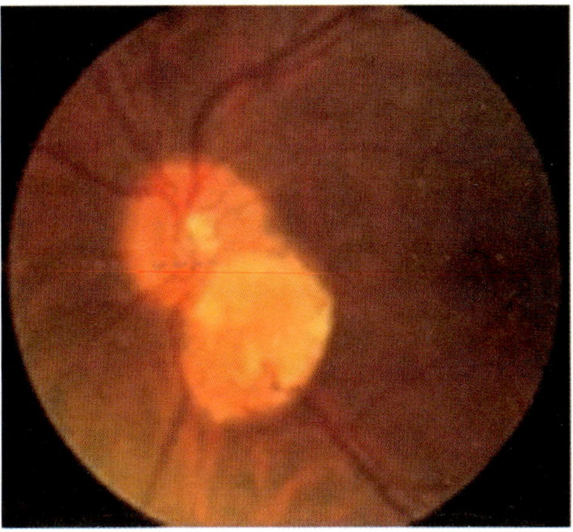

**Fig. 17.9**: Large multinodular retinal hamartoma

## 17.15. Corneal Clouding

Corneal clouding develops in: (FM3)

1. Mucopolysaccharidoses, all of which show corneal clouding, except MPSII and MPSIII.
2. Mucolipidoses.
3. Fucosidosis.
4. Mannosidosis.

## 17.16. Differential Diagnosis of Retinal Hemorrhages in an Infant with Suspected Shaking Injury (Not Exhaustive)

1. Nonaccidental shaking injury
2. Accidental injury (severe trauma)
3. Leukemia
4. Coagulation disorders
5. Birth hemorrhages
6. Meningococcal meningitis
7. Glutaric aciduria type I
8. Severe papilledema with raised intracranial pressure
9. Copper deficiency
10. Meningococcal meningitis.

### 17.17. Ophthalmological Photos

1. **Aniridia**: No iris tissue is seen. There is fibrovascular pannus covering the peripheral cornea in this case.

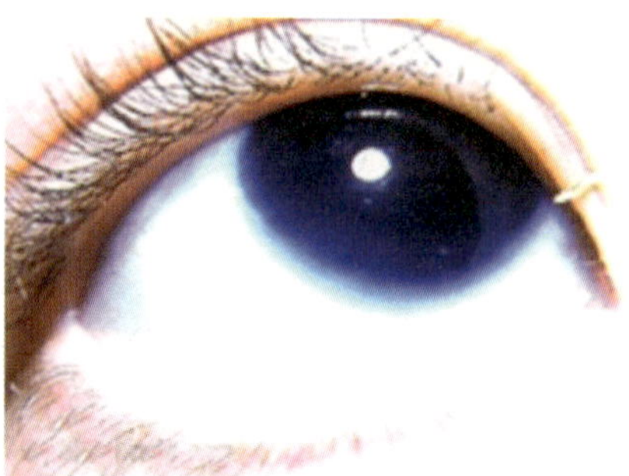

**Fig. 17.10**: Aniridia

2. **Coloboma of the inferior iris.**

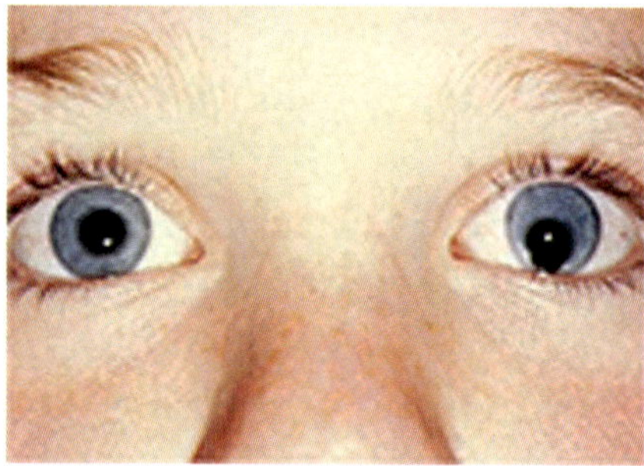

**Fig. 17.11**: Coloboma of inferior iris

3. **Iritis**: The pupil has been dilated and adhesions between the iris and lens (posterior synechiae) are seen.

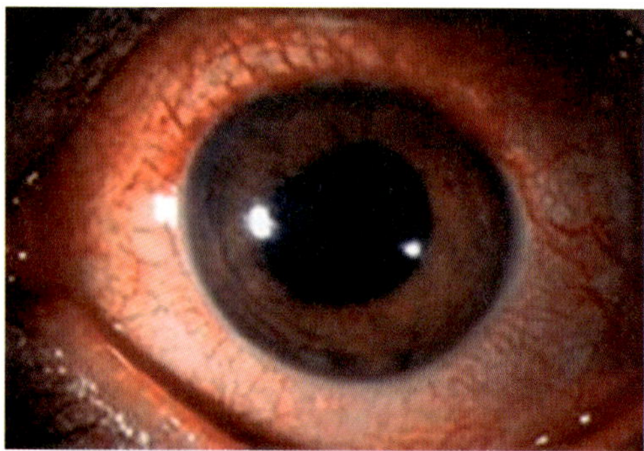

**Fig. 17.12**: Iritis

4. **Congenital cataract**: This is a partial, lamellar cataract with relatively good vision. Surgery in infancy was not needed in this case.

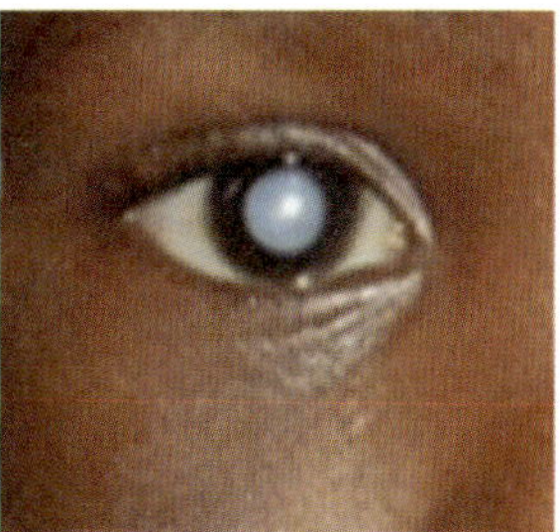

**Fig. 17.13**: Congenital cataract

5. **Subluxed lens.**

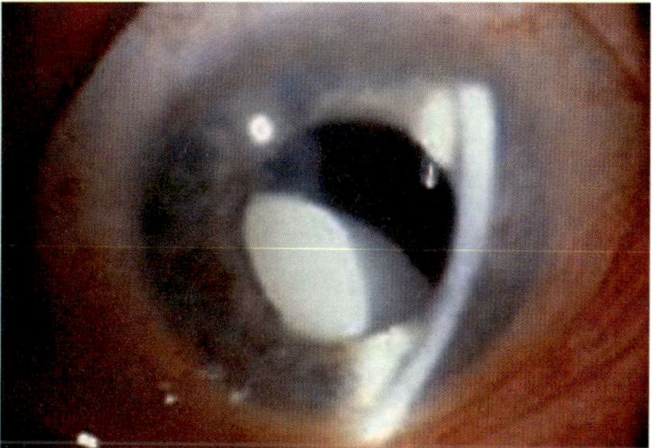

**Fig. 17.14**: Subluxation of the lens

6. **Reiger syndrome**: Note posterior embryotoxon and abnormal pupil shape and position (corectopia).

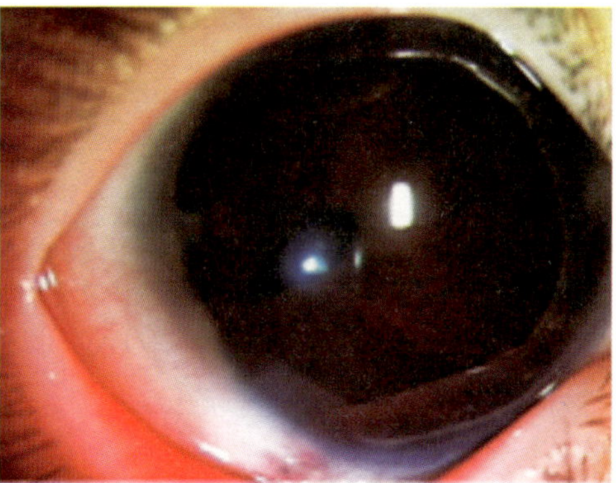

**Fig. 17.15**: Corectopia

7. **Sturge-Weber syndrome**: Note eyelid port wine stain, and abnormal scleral blood vessels.

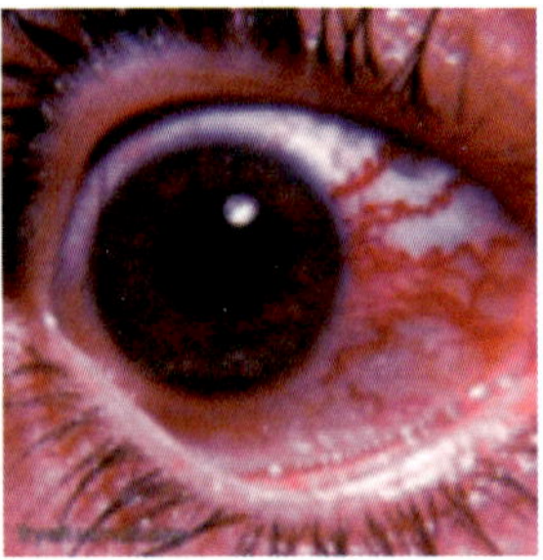

**Fig. 17.16**: Telangiectasia of the sclera

8. **Lisch nodules of the iris**: Multiple pigmented nodules are easily visualized against the background of a lightly pigmented iris in this case.

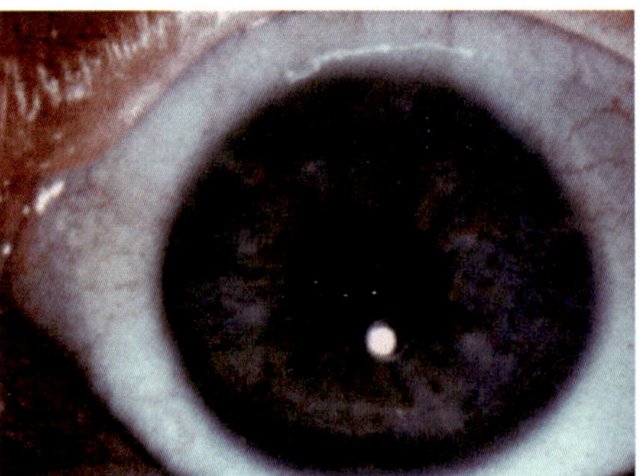

**Fig. 17.17**: Lisch nodules of the iris

9. **Hyphema**: Blood in the anterior chamber obscures the iris.

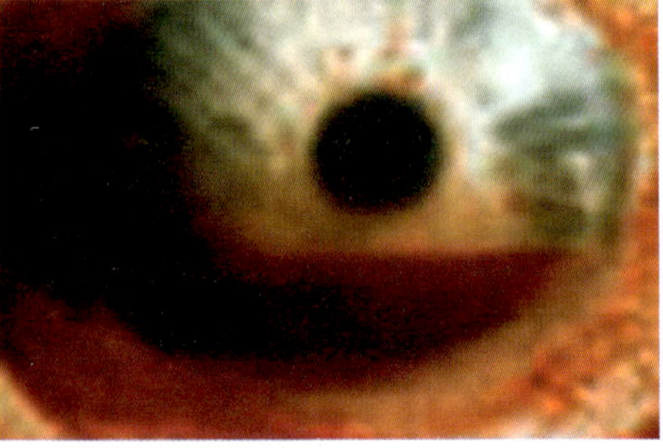

**Fig. 17.18**: Hyphema

10. **Retinoblastoma:** Inspection for a red reflex (Bruckner test) in this child revealed asymmetry with leukocoria (White pupil) of the right eye secondary to retinoblastoma.

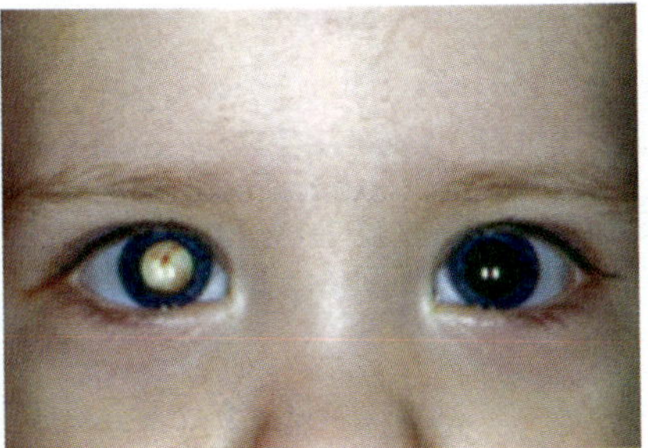

**Fig. 17.19:** Retinoblastoma

## 17.18. Stages of Papilledema (Frisen Scale)

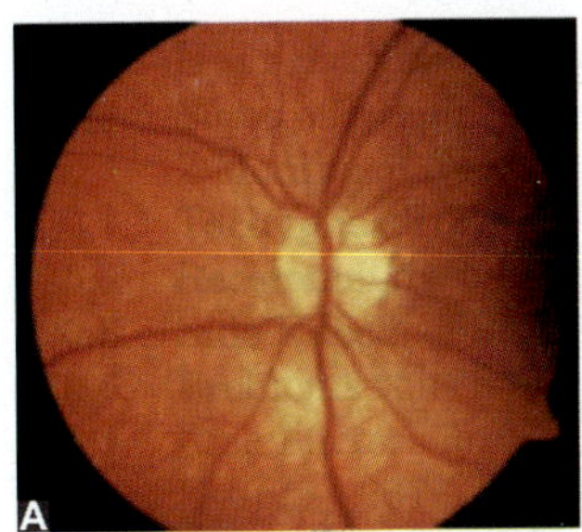

A. Stage 0: Normal optic disk.

B. Stage 1: Very early papilledema
  1. Obscuration of the nasal border of the disk only.
  2. Without elevation of the disk borders.

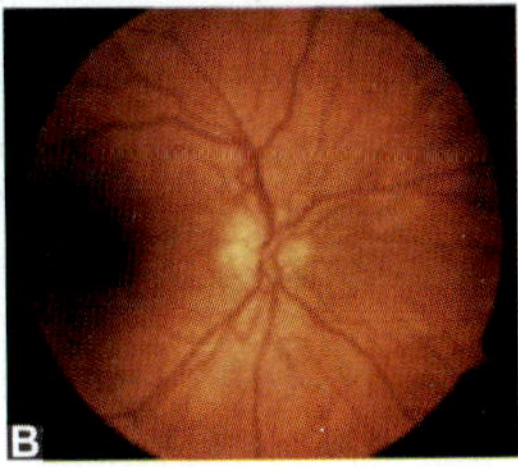

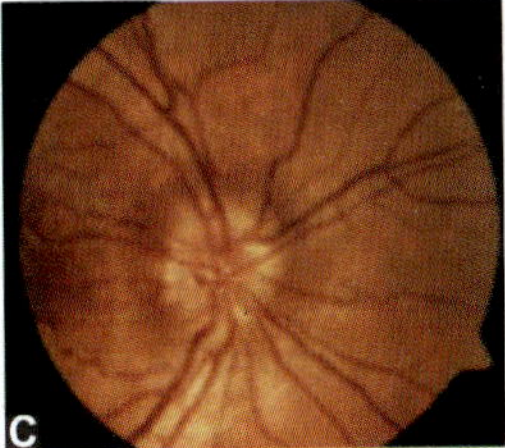

C. Stage 2: Early papilledema
  1. Obscuration of all borders
  2. Elevation of the nasal border
  3. Complete peripapillary halo.

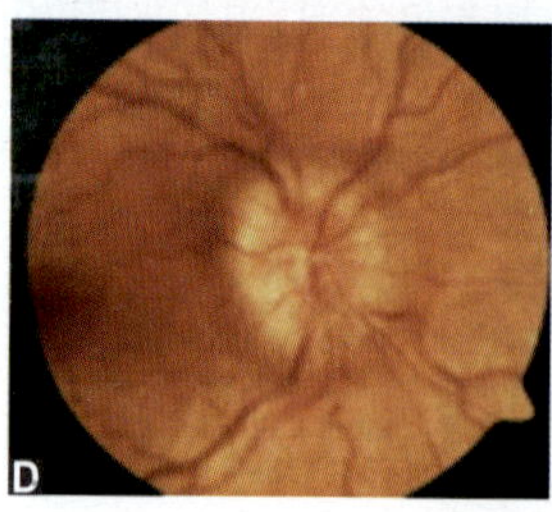

D. Stage 3: Moderate papilledema
1. Elevation of all borders.
2. Increased diameter of the optic nerve head.
3. Obscuration of vessels at the disk margin.
4. Peripapillary halo with finger-like extensions.

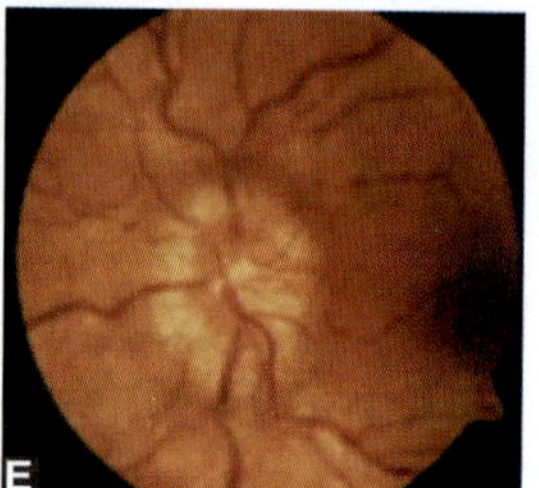

E. Stage 4: Marked papilledema
1. Elevation of the entire nerve head.
2. Total obscuration a segment of a major blood vessel on the disk.

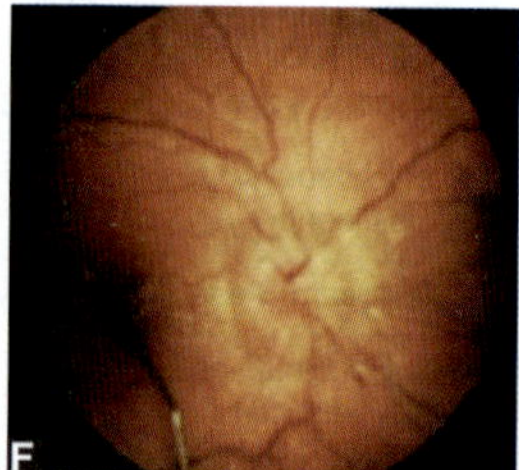

F. Stage 5: Severe papilledema
1. Obscuration of all vessels.
2. Obliteration of the optic cup.
3. Nerve fiber layer hemorrhages and macular exudate.

**Figs 17.20A to F**: Various stages of papilledema
(*Courtesy*: University of Rochester Eye Institute)

## Bibliography


1. http://content.lib.utah.edu/utils/getfile/collection/EHSL-Moran-Neuro-opth/id/140/filename/88.pdf
2. http://emedicine.medscape.com/article/1211159-overview
3. http://en.wikipedia.org/wiki/Lisch_nodule
4. http://health-7.com
5. http://imagebank.asrs.org
6. http://optometrist.com.au/children-cataracts/
7. http://webeye.ophth.uiowa.edu
8. http://webeye.ophth.uiowa.edu/eyeforum/cases-i/case114/DDX.html _
9. http://www.aapos.org/terms/conditions/82
10. http://www.aapos.org/terms/conditions/83

11. http://www.allaboutvision.com/conditions/congenital-cataracts.htm
12. http://www.beltina.org
13. http://www.gfmer.ch/genetic_diseases_v2/gendis_detail_list.php? cat3=2181
14. http://www.mrcophth.com/pd/oppticoa.html
15. http://www.nei.nih.gov/healthyeyestoolkit/factsheets/refractiveerrors.pdf
16. http://www.stlukeseye.com
17. http://www.varga.org/Physician%20Assistant%20Photos.htm
18. webeye.ophth.uiowa.edu
19. www.beautifulcanvas.org
20. www.lookfordiagnosis.com
21. www.willseye.org

# Orthopedic

## 18.1. Differential Diagnosis of Joint Pain in Children

### 18.1.1. Arthritis

1. Infective and reactive
2. Juvenile idiopathic arthritis
3. Other:
    i. Autoimmune rheumatic disorders, e.g.
        a. Systemic lupus erythematosus
        b. Dermatomyositis.
    ii. Vasculitis
    iii. Miscellaneous.

### 18.1.2. Mechanical/degenerative

1. Trauma: Accidental and nonaccidental.
2. Hypermobility.
3. Avascular necrosis, osteochondritis and apophysitis, including Perthes, Osgood-Schlatter and Scheuermann.
4. Slipped capital femoral epiphysis.
5. Anterior knee pain.

### 18.1.3. Nonorganic/idiopathic

1. Idiopathic pain syndromes—Localized and diffuse
2. Benign idiopathic limb pains (growing pains)
3. Psychogenic.

### 18.1.4. Other

1. Osteomyelitis.
2. Tumors:
    i. Malignant: Leukemia and neuroblastoma
    ii. Benign: Osteoid osteoma and pigmented villonodular synovitis.

3.  Metabolic abnormalities: Rickets, diabetes, hypophosphatemic rickets and hypo/hyperthyroidism.
4.  Genetic disorders: Skeletal dysplasias, mucopolysaccharidoses and collagen disorders.

## 18.2.  Hypermobility, Criteria Most Frequently Used to Define

The definition of hypermobility is based on clinical assessment. The criteria most frequently used are those defined by Beighton which assess joint laxity based on a number of clinical maneuvers:

1.  Passive dorsiflexion of the 5th metacarpophalangeal joint to 90°.
2.  Apposition of the thumb to the flexor aspect of the forearm.
3.  Hyperextension of the elbow to greater than 10°.
4.  Hyperextension of the knee to greater than 10°.
5.  Forward flexion of the trunk to place the palms of the hands flat on the floor with the knees extended.

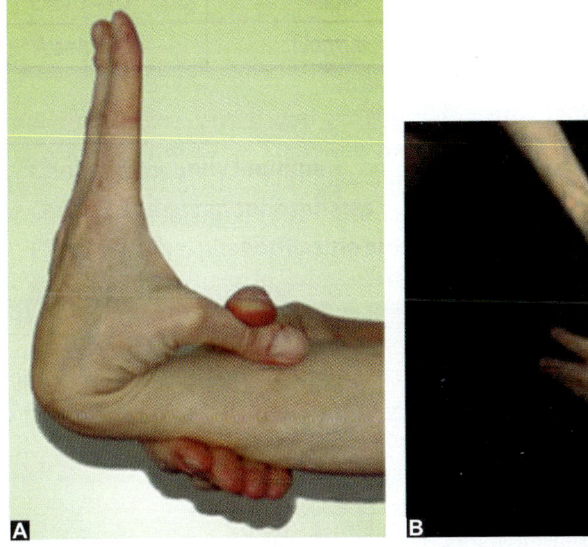 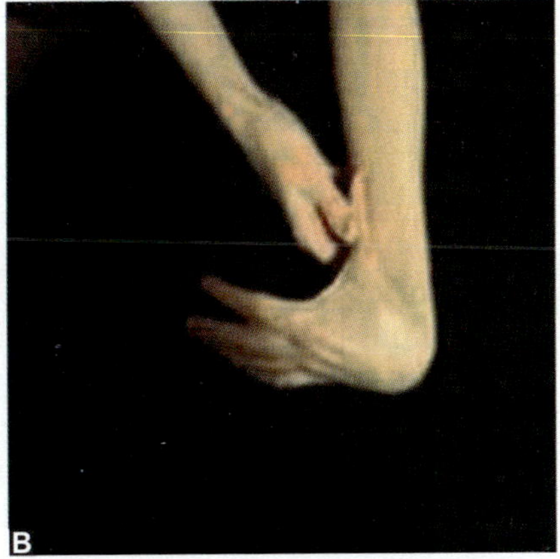

**Figs 18.1A and B**: Hypermobility: (A) Apposition of the thumb to the flexor aspect of the forearm (B) Extension of the thumb

## 18.3.  Inherited Syndromes with Significant Hypermobility

1.  Ehlers-Danlos syndrome
2.  Marfan syndrome
3.  Osteogenesis imperfecta
4.  Stickler syndrome.

## 18.4.　Inherited Skeletal Dysplasias

1.  Spondyloepiphyseal dysplasia (SED)
2.  Multiple epiphyseal dysplasia
3.  Achondroplasia and hypochondroplasia
4.  Trichorhinophalangeal dysplasia
5.  Storage disorders: The mucopolysaccharidoses (MPS).

## 18.5.　Differential Diagnosis of Inflammatory Arthritis in Childhood

1.  Infection—Differential diagnosis include:
    a.  Acute septic arthritis
    b.  Viral arthritis
    c.  Reactive/postinfectious arthritis.
2.  Juvenile idiopathic arthritis
    a.  The most common chronic rheumatologic disease in children
    b.  One of the most common chronic diseases of childhood
    c.  The etiology is unknown
    d.  The genetic component is complex.
3.  Arthritis associated with inflammatory bowel disease: Inflammatory bowel disease (IBD) refers to two disorders — Crohn's disease and ulcerative colitis arthritis associated with IBD.
    a.  Inflammation tends to involve only a few, large joints and it tends not to involve both sides of the body equally.
    b.  Antibodies commonly found in the blood of people with rheumatoid arthritis are not usually present in the blood of people with IBD arthritis.
    c.  Unlike rheumatoid arthritis, arthritis associated with IBD may affect the lower spine, specially the sacroiliac joints.
    d.  Is associated with a certain gene (called HLA-B27).
4.  Other autoimmune rheumatic disorders
    a.  Systemic lupus erythematosus
    b.  Juvenile dermatomyositis
    c.  Systemic sclerosis
    d.  Mixed connective tissue disease.
5.  Systemic vasculitis
    a.  Henoch-Schönlein purpura
    b.  Kawasaki disease
    c.  Polyarteritis nodosa.
6.  Malignancy
    a.  Leukemia
    b.  Neuroblastoma.

7. Hematological
   a. Sickle cell anemia
   b. Hemophilia.
8. Immune deficiency syndromes
9. Genetic disorders
   a. Cystic fibrosis
   b. Velocardiofacial syndrome
   c. CINCA syndrome
   d. Down syndrome
   e. Stickler syndrome.
   CINCA: Chronic infantile neurological cutaneous and articular syndrome .
10. Drug reactions
11. Trauma including nonaccidental injury
12. Orthopedic
    a. Perthes disease
    b. Pigmented villonodular synovitis.
13. Miscellaneous
    a. Sarcoidosis
    b. SAPHO syndrome
    c. Familial mediterranean fever.
    SAPHO: Synovitis, acne, pustulosis, hyperostosis and osteitis syndrome .

## 18.6. The Differential Diagnosis of Joint Pain in Children

### 18.6.1. Arthritis

- Infective and reactive.
- Juvenile idiopathic arthritis.
- Other: Autoimmune rheumatic disorders (e.g. systemic lupus erythematosus and dermatomyositis); vasculitis; miscellaneous.

### 18.6.2. Mechanical/degenerative

- Trauma: Accidental and nonaccidental.
- Hypermobility.
- Avascular necrosis, osteochondritis and apophysitis, including Perthes, Osgood-Schlatter and Scheuermann.
- Slipped capital femoral epiphysis.
- Anterior knee pain.

### 18.6.3. Nonorganic/idiopathic

- Idiopathic pain syndromes—Localized and diffuse
- Benign idiopathic limb pains (growing pains)
- Psychogenic.

### 18.6.4. Other

- Osteomyelitis.
- Malignant tumors: Leukemia and neuroblastoma.
- Benign: Osteoid osteoma and pigmented villonodular synovitis.
- Metabolic abnormalities: Rickets, diabetes, hypophosphatemic rickets and hypo/hyperthyroidism.
- Genetic disorders: Skeletal dysplasias, mucopolysaccharidoses and collagen disorders.

## 18.7. Comparison of Synovial Fluid Analysis in Children with Infective and Inflammatory Arthritis

| Characteristic | Normal | Juvenile idiopathic arthritis | Septic arthritis |
|---|---|---|---|
| Color | Yellow | Yellow | Serosanguinous |
| Clarity | Clear | Cloudy | Turbid |
| WBC count/mm$^3$ | < 200 | $15–20 \times 10^3$ | $40–300000 \times 10^3$ |
| PMN count (%) | < 25 | 60–75 | > 75 |
| PMN—Polymorphic neutrophil, WBC—White blood cell | | | |

## 18.8. Psoriatic Arthritis

Psoriatic arthritis is defined as arthritis and psoriasis, or arthritis and at least two of the following:
- Dactylitis
- Nail pitting and onycholysis
- Psoriasis in a first-degree relative.

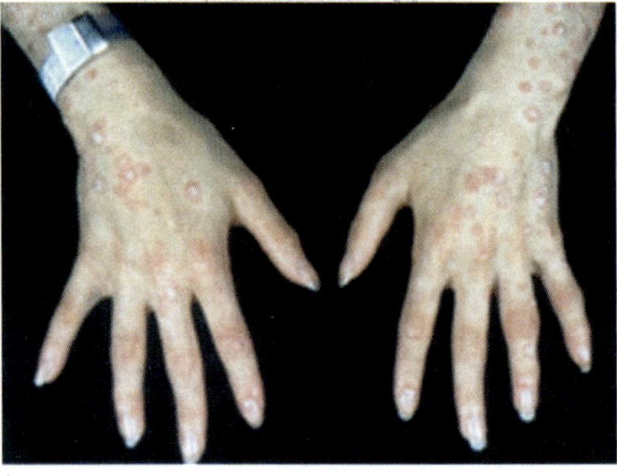

**Fig. 18.2:** Psoriatic arthritis

## 18.9.   Criteria for the Diagnosis of Rheumatic Fever

| Modified Jones criteria for the diagnosis of rheumatic fever | |
|---|---|
| **Major criteria** | **Minor criteria** |
| Polyarthritis (common): Flitting and large joints | Fever |
| Carditis (common): Pancarditis | Arthralgia |
| Chorea (Sydenham) (uncommon): Persistent | Prolonged P-R interval |
| Erythema marginatum (uncommon): Macules evolving to serpiginous | Elevated ESR/CRP, leukocytosis |
| Subcutaneous nodules (uncommon): Extensor surfaces | Previous rheumatic fever |

The diagnosis of rheumatic fever is made in the presence of either two major criteria or one major plus two minor criteria together with evidence of recent group A streptococcal infection:

  i.   Positive throat swab

  ii.  Elevated antistreptolysin O titer (ASOT)

  iii. Other antistreptococcal antibodies.

## 18.10.  Roles of Radiological Imaging in Juvenile Idiopathic Arthritis (JIA)

### 18.10. 1.   All imaging modalities may have a potential role in JIA to

- Aid diagnosis—Particularly to exclude other musculoskeletal conditions.
- Document and define evidence of joint damage.
- Aid the assessment of complex joints, e.g. hip, subtalar, shoulder and temporomandibular joints.
- Detect subclinical or very early synovitis—Magnetic resonance scanning with gadolinium contrast is a very sensitive technique.
- Distinguish synovitis from tenosynovitis.
- Facilitate intra-articular steroid injection.

### 18.10. 2.  Stages of radiographic changes are seen on plain radiographs in JIA are 3

- **Early**: Soft tissue swelling, e.g. blurring of the infrapatellar fat pad on lateral knee radiograph and periarticular osteopenia.
- **Intermediate**: Cortical erosions, joint space narrowing and subchondral cysts.
- **Late**: Destructive joint changes with ankylosis, joint contractures, metaphyseal and diaphyseal changes and growth anomalies.

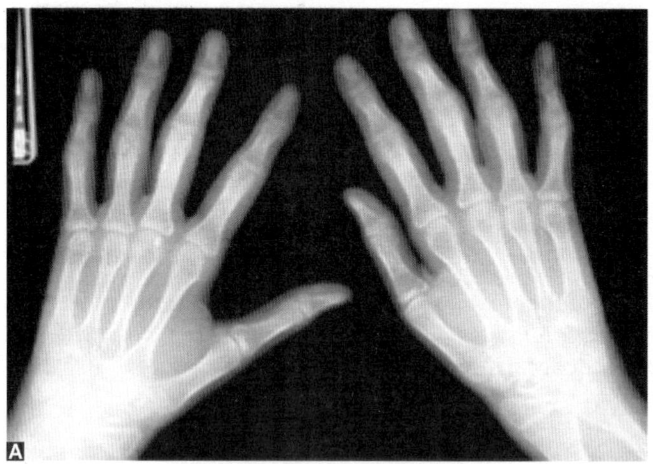

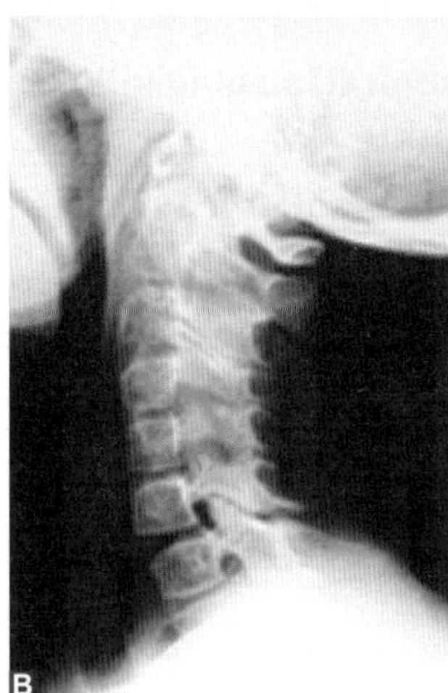

Plain radiographs in juvenile idiopathic arthritis: (A) Destructive changes of wrists with crowding of carpal bones; periarticular osteopenia and loss of joint space at proximal interphalangeal joints; (B) Fusion in block of posterior elements of C2–C7

**Fig. 18.3**: Radiography for juvenile idiopathic arthritis

## 18.11. Kawasaki Disease

**Diagnostic criteria for Kawasaki disease**

Fever persisting for at least 5 days plus four of the following features:

1. Changes in peripheral extremities or perineal area
2. Polymorphous exanthema
3. Bilateral conjunctival injection
4. Changes of lips and oral/pharyngeal mucosa
5. Cervical lymphadenopathy.

In the presence of confirmed coronary artery involvement and fever, less than four of the remaining criteria are sufficient to make the diagnosis.

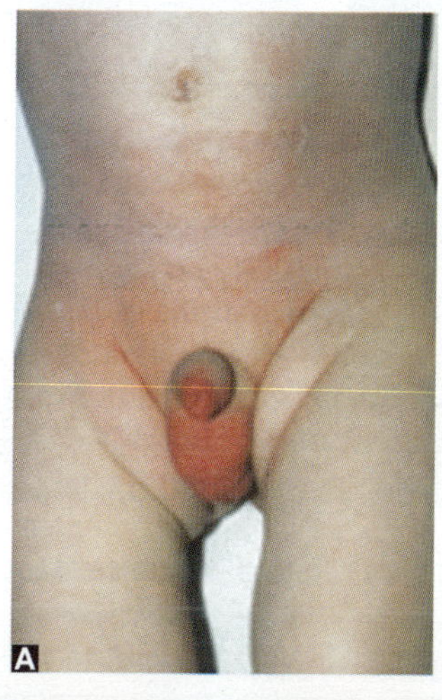

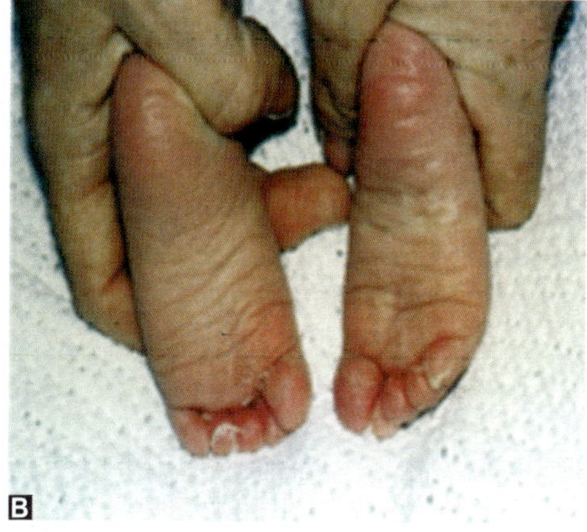

**Figs 18.4A and B**: Kawasaki disease. A: Typical erythematous groin rash with peeling and B: Peeling of digits

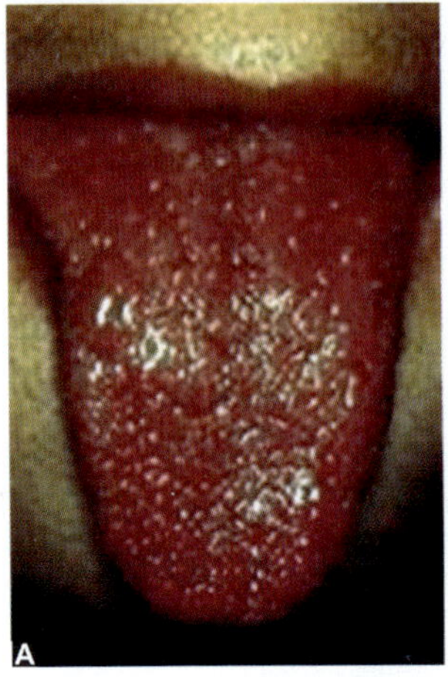

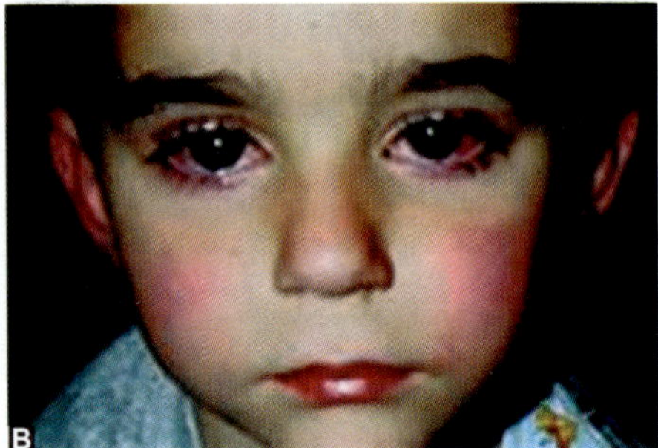

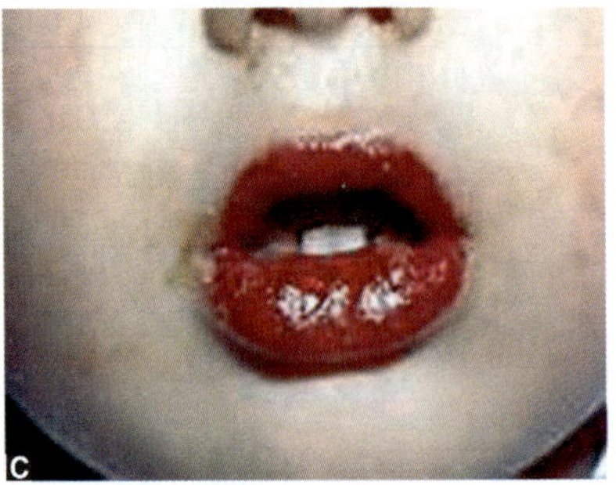

**Figs 18.5A to C**: Kawasaki disease

## 18.12. Juvenile Dermatomyositis

| Diagnostic criteria for Juvenile Dermatomyositis | |
| --- | --- |
| Classic rash | Heliotrope rash of the eyelids<br>Gottron papules |
| Plus three of the following: | |
| Weakness | Symmetric<br>Proximal |
| Muscle enzyme elevation (≥1) | Creatine kinase<br>Aspartate aminotransferase<br>Lactate dehydrogenase<br>aldolase |
| Electromyographic changes | Myopathy<br>Denervation |
| Muscle biopsy | Necrosis<br>Inflammation |

## 18.13. Systemic Lupus Erythematosus

1. Malar rash
2. Discoid rash
3. Photosensitivity
4. Serositis:
   a. Pleuritis
   b. Pericarditis.
5. Arthritis
6. Hematological disorders:
   a. Hemolytic anemia
   b. Leukopenia < 4× 109/L (two or more occasions)
   c. Lymphopenia < 1.5109/L (two or more occasions)
   d. Thrombocytopenia < 100 × 109/L.
7. Immunological disorders:
   a. Raised antinative DNA antibody binding
   b. Anti-Sm antibody
   c. Antiphospholipid antibodies:
      i. Abnormal serum levels of IgG or IgM anticardiolipin antibodies.
      ii. Positive test for lupus anticoagulant.
      iii. False-positive serological test for syphilis  present for at least 3 months.
8. Oral ulceration.
9. Renal disorder:
   a. Proteinuria > 0.5 gm/24 hours
   b. Cellular casts.
10. Neurological disorder:
    a. Seizures
    b. Psychosis (other causes excluded).
11. Antinuclear antibody present in raised titer.

A person shall be said to have SLE if four or more of the 11 criteria are present (serially or simultaneously).

## Bibliography


1. http://emedicine.medscape.com/article/1417215-overview
2. http://himho.com/kawasaki-disease
3. http://www.aafp.org/afp/2006/0701/p115.html
4. http://www.arthritis.org/conditions-treatments/disease-center/juvenile—arthritis
5. http://www.cdc.gov/arthritis/basics/childhood.htm
6. http://www.medicinenet.com/hypermobility_syndrome/article.htm

7. http://www.ncbi.nlm.nih.gov/pmc/articles/PMC1311464/
8. http://www.niams.nih.gov/Health_Info/Lupus/default.asp
9. http://www.pediatriconcall.com/m/doctor/DiseasesandCondition/PEDIATRIC_CARDIOLOGY/diagnosis.asp
10. www.rheumatology.org/practice/clinical/patients/diseases_and_conditions/psoriaticarthritis.asp

# Otolaryngology

## 19.1. Facts about ENT

### 19.1.1. Facts about ears

1. 95% of traumatic tympanic membrane perforations will close spontaneously and return to normal.
2. Acute otitis media is the most common cause of otalgia with fever in children.
3. Postaural subperiosteal swelling with a protruding pinna is pathognomonic of acute mastoiditis.
4. Otitis media with effusion is the most common cause of conductive deafness in childhood.
5. Surgery for otitis media with effusion should only follow 3 months of watchful waiting.
6. Significant bilateral sensorineural deafness has an incidence of one in 1000 live births.
7. Only about 50% of children with significant bilateral sensorineural loss have an identifiable cause.
8. Early diagnosis of sensorineural deafness is vital for acquisition of speech and language.
9. Only 50% of children with sensorineural deafness have an identifiable cause.
10. Cochlear implants are only required for a very small number of profoundly deaf children.

### 19.1.2. Facts about nose

1. Unilateral foul-smelling nasal discharge in a young child is pathognomonic of a nasal foreign body.
2. Epistaxis in a child usually comes from Little's area at the front of the nose and can be controlled by local pressure.
3. Periorbital infection often arises from infection of the ethmoid or frontal sinuses and should be treated vigorously.
4. Gasping respiration in a neonate is suggestive of choanal atresia.

### 19.1.3. Facts about Tonsils

1.  There is no good evidence that antibiotics for tonsillitis alter the course or severity of the acute episode.

## 19.2.    Causes of Sensorineural Deafness

### 19.2.1. Prenatal causes

#### *19.2.1.1. Hereditary causes*

1.  Waardenburg syndrome
2.  Klippel-Feil syndrome
3.  Alport syndrome
4.  Pendred syndrome
5.  Refsum syndrome
6.  Usher syndrome
7.  Jervell and Lange-Nielsen syndrome.

#### *19.2.1.2. Nonhereditary causes*

- Maternal illness, specially in the first trimester of pregnancy:
    1.  Cytomegalovirus infections
    2.  Toxoplasmosis
    3.  Glandular fever
    4.  Rubella.
- Ototoxic drugstaking during pregnancy:
    1.  Aminoglycosides
    2.  Quinine
    3.  Salicylates
    4.  Alcohol.

### 19.2.2. Perinatal causes

1.  Prematurity
2.  Hypoxia.

### 19.2.3. Postnatal causes

1.  Head injury
2.  Ototoxic drugs
3.  Specific infections:
    – Measles
    – Mumps
    – Meningococcal or pneumococcal meningitis.

## 19.3.  Symptoms of Sensorineural Deafness

### 19.3.1.  Sensorineural deafness is hearing loss that occurs from damage to

1.  The inner ear
2.  Auditory nerve
3.  The brain.

### 19.3.2.  Symptoms may include

- Certain sounds seem too loud
- Difficulty following conversations when two or more people are talking
- Difficulty hearing in noisy areas
- Easier to hear men's voices than women's voices
- Hard to tell high-pitched sounds (such as "s" or "th") from one another
- Other people's voices sound mumbled or slurred
- Problems hearing when there is background noise.

## 19.4.  Common Causes of Stridor in Infants and Children

a.  **Nose**: Choanal atresia in newborn
b.  **Tongue**:
    i.  Macroglossia due to cretinism
    ii.  Hemangioma or lymphangioma and dermoid at base of tongue
    iii.  Lingual thyroid.
c.  **Mandible**
    i.  Micrognathia
    ii.  Pierre-Robin syndrome.
d.  **Pharynx**
    i.  Congenital dermoid
    ii.  Adenotonsillar hypertrophy
    iii.  Retropharyngeal abscess and tumors.
e.  **Larynx**
    i.  Congenital:
        1.  Laryngeal web
        2.  Laryngomalacia
        3.  Cysts
        4.  Vocal cord paralysis
        5.  Subglottic stenosis.
    ii.  Inflammatory:
        1.  Epiglottitis
        2.  Laryngotracheitis

       3. Diphtheria

       4. Tuberculosis.

  iii. Neoplastic

       1. Hemangioma

       2. Juvenile multiple papillomas.

  iv. Traumatic:

       1. Injuries of larynx

       2. Foreign bodies

       3. Edema following endoscopy

       4. Prolonged intubation.

   v. Miscellaneous:

       1. Tetanus

       2. Tetany

       3. Laryngismus stridulus.

  vi. Neurogenic: Laryngeal paralysis due to acquired lesions.

**f. Trachea and bronchi**

   i. Congenital:

       1. Atresia

       2. Stenosis

       3. Tracheomalacia.

   ii. Inflammatory: Tracheobronchitis.

  iii. Traumatic:

       1. Foreign body

       2. Stenosis trachea.

  iv. Neoplastic: Tumors of trachea.

**g. Lesions outside respiratory tract**

   i. Congenital:

       1. Vascular rings

       2. Esophageal atresia

       3. Tracheoesophageal fistula

       4. Congenital goiter

       5. Cystic hygroma.

   ii. Inflammatory: Retropharyngeal and retroesophageal abscess.

  iii. Traumatic: Foreign body esophagus.

  iv. Tumors: Masses in neck.

## 19.5. Normal CT Scan for the Paranasal Sinuses

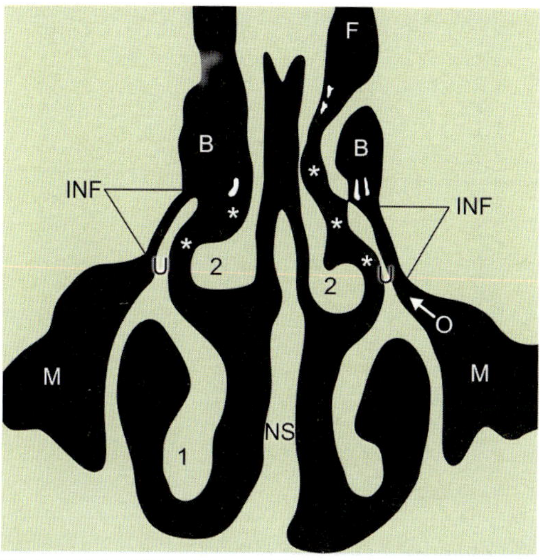


Ostiomeatal unit line drawing: Inferior turbinate (1) middle turbinate (2) maxillary sinus (M), uncinate (U), ethmoidal bulla (B), mrontal sinus (F), ethmoidal infundibulum (INF), nasal septum (NS) and middle meatus (*)

**Fig. 19.1**: CT scan of normal paranasal sinuses

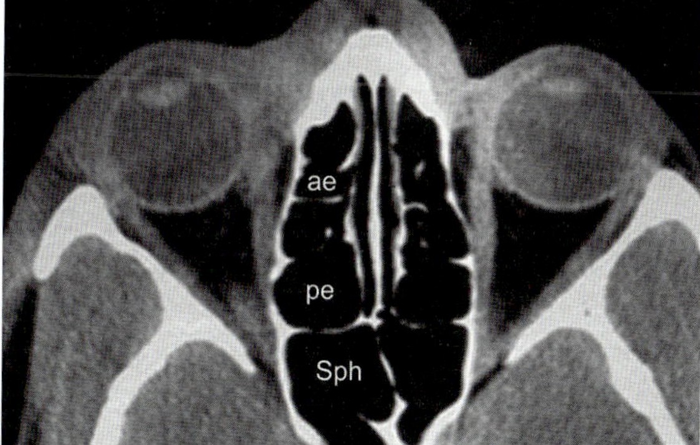


Axial images of the anterior (ae) and posterior (pe) ethmoid air cells. The sphenoid sinus (Sph) can be seen with its intersinus septum

**Fig. 19.2**: CT scan of normal paranasal sinuses

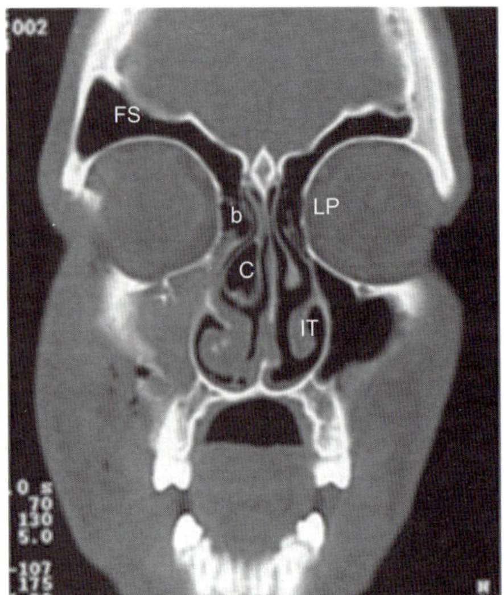

Coronal view demonstrating well-pneumatized frontal sinuses (FS), the ethmoid bulla (b), and the lamina papyracea (LP). Also of interest is the presence of an aerated middle turbinate or concha bullosa (C) blocking the ostiomeatal complex. The inferior turbinate is labeled IT

**Fig. 19.3**: Coronal view for the sinuses

## 19.6.  Lateral Soft Tissue X-ray of a 4-year-old Boy

Showing enlarged adenoids occluding the postnasal airway (arrowed).

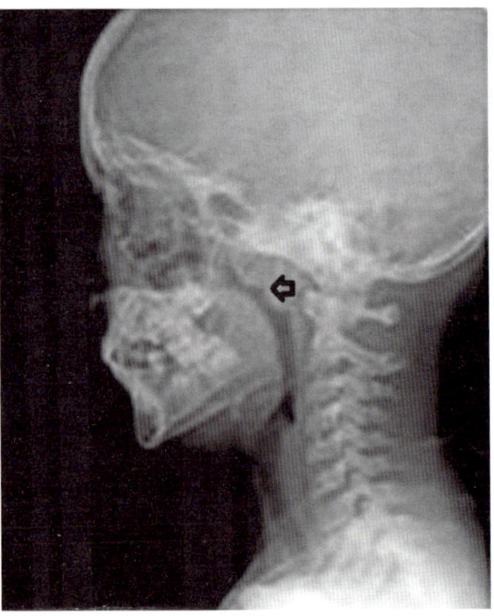

**Fig. 19.4**: Lateral soft X-ray

## 19.7. Adenoidectomy

### 19.7.1. Indications

- Persistent mouth breathing.
- Repeated or chronic otitis media with effusion.
- Hyponasal speech.
- Adenoid facies.
- Persistent or recurrent nasopharyngitis when it seems to be temporarily related to hypertrophied adenoid tissue.

### 19.7.2. Fact

Tonsillectomy is NOT performed for those above problems.

## 19.8. Tonsillectomy

### 19.8.1. Indications

- Recurrent pharyngitis:
  - 7 episodes in the past year
  - 5 in each of the last 2 years
  - 3 in each of the past 3 years.
- Marked severe adenotonsillar hypertrophy
- Severe sleep apnea.

### 19.8.2. Facts

- Tonsillectomy does NOT help with preventing or treating acute or chronic sinusitis or chronic otitis media.
- Tonsillectomy does NOT help preventing UTIs.

## 19.9.   Causes of Hoarseness in Children

The causes of hoarseness in children
1. Vocal nodules
2. Polyps of the larynx
3. Laryngeal papillomas
4. Unilateral vocal cord paralysis.

### 19.9.1.  Laryngeal diagnoses of the causes of hoarseness in children

1. Reflux laryngitis
2. True vocal fold nodules
3. Laryngomalacia.

## 19.10. Complications of Tonsillitis

- Peritonsillitis
- Peritonsillar abscess (quinsy)
- Airway obstruction
- Rheumatic fever and glomerulonephritis.

### 19.10.1. Complications specific to group A β-hemolytic *Streptococcus pyogenes* (GABHS) pharyngitis

- Scarlet fever
- Rheumatic fever
- Septic arthritis
- Glomerulonephritis.

## 19.11. The Most Common Causes of Epistaxis in Children

### 19.11.1. Local causes

- Epistaxis digitorum (nose picking)
- Foreign bodies
- Trauma including child abuse
- Rhinitis
- Chronic sinusitis.

### 19.11.2. Nasal causes

- Intranasal neoplasm or polyps
- Septal deviation
- Septal perforation
- Vascular malformation or telangiectasia.

### 19.11.3. Blood diseases

- Hemophilia
- Platelet dysfunction
- Thrombocytopenia
- Hypertension
- Leukemia.

### 19.11.4. Other causes

- Liver disease (e.g. cirrhosis).
- Medications (e.g. aspirin, anticoagulants, nonsteroidal anti-inflammatory drugs and topical corticosteroids).

## 19.12. Serous Otitis Media (Secretory Otitis Media)

### 19.12.1. Causes of serous otitis media

1.  Malfunctioning of eustachian tube:
    - i.   Adenoid hyperplasia
    - ii.  Chronic rhinitis and sinusitis
    - iii. Chronic tonsillitis
    - iv.  Palatal defects.
2.  Allergy
3.  Unresolved otitis media
4.  Viral infections.

### 19.12.2. Symptoms of serous otitis media

- i.   Hearing loss
- ii.  Delayed and defective speech
- iii. Mild earaches.

## 19.13. Predisposing Factors for Acute Suppurative Otitis Media

1.  Recurrent attacks of common cold, upper respiratory tract infections and exanthematous fevers like measles, diphtheria and whooping cough.
2.  Infections of tonsils and adenoids.
3.  Chronic rhinitis and sinusitis.
4.  Nasal allergy.
5.  Tumors of nasopharynx, packing of nose or nasopharynx for epistaxis.
6.  Cleft palate.

## Bibliography


1. http://earnosethroatclinic.blogspot.ae/2010/12/stridor-causes-and-differential.html
2. http://emedicine.medscape.com/article/871977-clinical
3. http://emedicine.medscape.com/article/875244-overview#a16
4. http://oto.sagepub.com/
5. http://radiopaedia.org/articles/adenoids-1
6. http://www.emedicinehealth.com/nosebleeds/page2_em.htm#nosebleed_causes
7. http://www.entusa.com/tonsillectomy_surgery.htm
8. http://www.medscape.com/viewarticle/433482
9. http://www.nlm.nih.gov/medlineplus/ency/article/003291.htm

# Respiratory Disorders

## 20.1. The AAP Guidelines for RSV Immunoprophylaxis for High-risk Infants and Children

1. Infants and children <24 months with chronic lung disease of prematurity who require medical therapy (e.g. diuretics  oxygen) within 6 months before the start of RSV season.
2. Infants born at <32 weeks gestation at the start of RSV season, those born at 29–32 weeks benefit most upto 6 months of age.
3. Infants born at <28 weeks gestation during the first months of life.
4. Children <24 months of age with hemodynamically significant cyanotic and acyanotic congenital heart disease.

   (NOT secundum ASD, small VSD, pulmonary stenosis, uncomplicated aortic stenosis, PDA, mild coarctation, or those with more severe disease who have been corrected and no longer require medication).
5. For those 32–35 weeks of age and with one of the following:
   - Attends day care
   - Infant has a sibling <5 years of age.

## 20.2. Signs of Respiratory Distress in an Infant Older than 2 Months of Age

- Tachypnea
- Subcostal retractions
- Cough
- Crackles
- Decreased breath sounds.

## 20.3. Tachypnea Thresholds based on Age—A Comparison

| Age | Normal (breaths/minute) | Tachypnea (breaths/minute) |
|---|---|---|
| 2–12 months | 25–40 | 50 |
| 1–5 years | 20–30 | 40 |
| > 5  years | 15–25 | 20 |

## 20.4.  Recommendations of Chest X-ray for Chest Infection

- Children under 5 years of age with fever and high WBCs of unknown source.
- There is clinical evidence of possible pneumonia, but the clinical findings are not clear-cut.
- Pleural effusion is suspected.
- Pneumonia is unresponsive to antibiotics.

## 20.5.  Side Effects of Systemic Corticosteroids

- Suppression of the hypothalamic-pituitary-adrenal axis
- Osteoporosis
- Cataracts
- Hypoglycemia
- Weight gain
- Thinning of the skin
- Striae
- Growth retardation.

## 20.6.  Problems that may be Caused by the Usage of Inhaled Steroids

- Growth velocity changes.
- Dermal thinning and increased ease of skin bruising.
- Rarely cataracts may form and hypothalamic-pituitary—Adrenal axis function may be affected.
- Oral candidiasis (thrush) is common.

## 20.7.  Risk Factors for Poor Prognosis in Drowning and Submersion Events Include

- Submersion >10 minutes
- >10 minutes elapsed before life support is begun at the scene
- Resuscitation takes >25 minutes
- Age <3 years
- Water temperature >10°C (50°F).

## 20.8.  Reasons to Consider Sweat Test

### 20.8.1. GI pearls for testing

- Meconium ileus
- Rectal prolapsed

- Prolonged neonatal jaundice
- Chronic diarrhea
- Steatorrhea.

### 20.8.2. Respiratory pearls for testing

- Nasal polyps
- Pansinusitis
- Chronic cough
- Recurrent wheezing
- *Staphylococcus aureus pneumonia*
- Finding *Pseudomonas* in throat, sputum, or bronchus cultures.

### 20.8.3. Miscellaneous pearls for testing

- Digital clubbing
- Family history of cystic fibrosis (CF)
- Failure to thrive (FTT)
- "My baby tastes salty"
- Male infertility.

## 20.9.  Hemoptysis in Children

### 20.9.1.  The most common etiologies in children are

- Infection
- Foreign bodies
- Bronchiectasis.

### 20.9.2.  Rare causes include

| Vascularitides: | Neoplasm |
| --- | --- |
| • HSP | AV malformation |
| • Wegener's | Hemangioma |
| • Goodpasture's | Trauma |
| • SLE | Pulmonary embolism |
| Congenital heart and lung defects | Idiopathic |

## 20.10. Sarcoidosis

### 20.10.1.  Indications for systemic corticosteroids in sarcoidosis

- Eyes involvement
- Heart conduction abnormalities

- CNS involvement
- Severe pulmonary symptoms
- Severe skin lesions
- Persistent hypercalcemia.

## 20.10.2. Radiological staging of sarcoidosis

| Stage | Chest X-ray findings |
|---|---|
| 0 | Clear |
| I | Bilateral hilar adenopathy |
| II | Adenopathy + parenchymal infiltrates |
| III | Diffuse parenchymal infiltrates |
| IV | Fibrosis, bullae and cavities |

## 20.10.3. Facts concerning sarcoidosis

- Erythema nodosum is an associated skin lesion that denotes a good prognosis.
- Corticosteroids have not been proven to induce remissions in sarcoidosis, although they do decrease the symptoms and pulmonary function tests.

## 20.10.4. Dermatologic manifestations of sarcoidosis

Dermatologic manifestations may include the following:
- Erythema nodosum.
- A lower-extremity panniculitis with painful, erythematous nodules (often with Löfgren syndrome).
- Lupus pernio (the most specific associated cutaneous lesion).
- Violaceous rash on the cheeks or nose (common).
- Maculopapular plaques (uncommon).

## 20.10.5. Laboratory evaluation of sarcoidosis

Routine laboratory evaluation is often unrevealing, but possible abnormalities include the following:
- Hypercalcemia (about 10–13% of patients)
- Hypercalciuria (about a third of patients)
- Elevated alkaline phosphatase level
- Elevated angiotensin-converting enzyme (ACE) levels.

## 20.11. Conditions Predisposing to Aspiration Lung Injury in Children

### 20.11.1. Anatomical and mechanical conditions

| | |
|---|---|
| Tracheoesophageal fistula | Esophageal foreign body |
| Laryngeal cleft | Tracheostomy |
| Vascular ring | Endotracheal tube |
| Cleft palate | Nasoenteric tube |
| Micrognathia | Collagen vascular disease (scleroderma and dermatomyositis) |
| Macroglossia | Gastroesophageal reflux disease |
| Achalasia | Obesity |

### 20.11.2. Neuromuscular conditions

| | |
|---|---|
| Altered consciousness | Muscular dystrophy |
| Immaturity of swallowing/prematurity | Myasthenia gravis |
| Dysautonomia | Guillain-Barré syndrome |
| Increased intracranial pressure | Werdnig-Hoffmann disease |
| Hydrocephalus | Ataxia-telangiectasia |
| Vocal cord paralysis | Cerebral vascular accident |
| Cerebral palsy | |

### 20.11.3. Miscellaneous

| | |
|---|---|
| Poor oral hygiene | Poor feeding techniques (bottle propping, overfeeding, inappropriate foods for toddlers) |
| Gingivitis | Bronchopulmonary dysplasia |
| Prolonged hospitalization | Viral infection |
| Gastric outlet or intestinal obstruction | |

## 20.12. Finger Clubbing

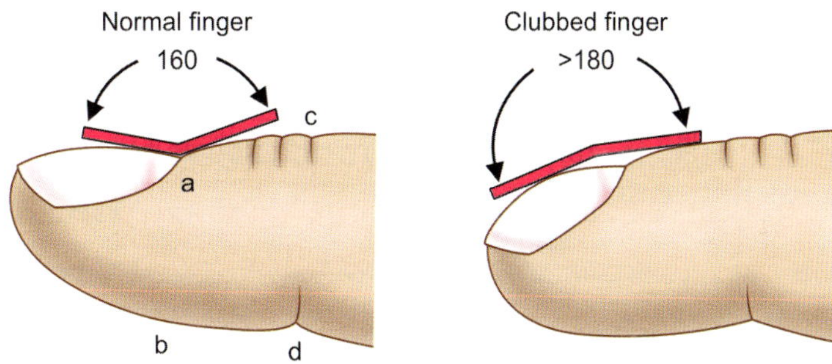



**Fig. 20.1**: Finger clubbing

## 20.12.1. Nonpulmonary diseases associated with clubbing

### 20.12.1.1. Cardiac diseases

1. Cyanotic congenital heart disease
2. Subacute bacterial endocarditis
3. Chronic congestive heart failure.

### 20.12.1.2. Hematological diseases

1. Thalassemia
2. Congenital methemoglobinemia (rare).

### 20.12.1.3. Gastrointestinal diseases

1. Ulcerative colitis
2. Chronic dysentery and sprue
3. Polyposis coli
4. Severe gastrointestinal hemorrhage
5. Small bowel lymphoma
6. Liver cirrhosis (including $\alpha_1$-antitrypsin deficiency).

### 20.12.1.4.  Other diseases

1. Thyroid deficiency (thyroid acropachy)
2. Chronic pyelonephritis (rare)
3. Toxic (e.g. arsenic, mercury and beryllium)
4. Lymphomatoid granulomatosis
5. Fabry disease
   - Raynaud disease and scleroderma.

## 20.13. Spirogram Showing Lung Volumes and Capacities

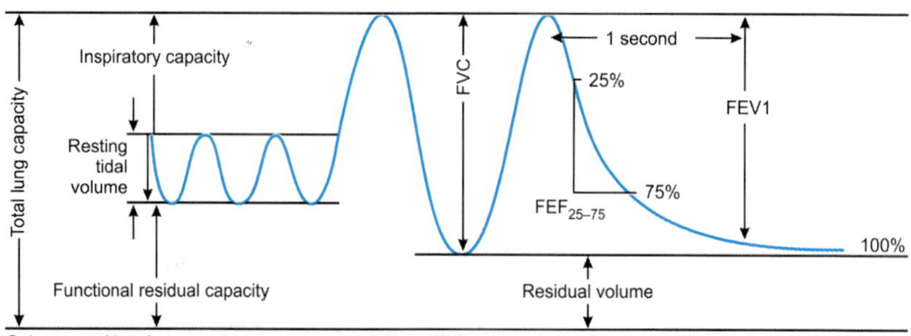


Spirogram with volumes and measurements. FEF 25–75, forced expiratory flow at 25–75% vital capacity; FEV1, forced expiratory volume in 1 second; FVC, forced vital capacity. (Adapted from Siberry GK, Iannone R (eds) The Johns Hopkins Hospital Harriet Lane Handbook, 15th ed. st. Louis: Mosby, 1999)

FEV1.0 is the maximum volume exhaled in 1 sec after maximum inspiration, FEV, forced expiratory volume

**Fig. 20.2**: Spirogram

- Restrictive diseases are usually associated with decreased lung volumes and capacities.
- Intrathoracic airway obstruction is associated with air trapping and abnormally high functional residual capacity and residual volume.
- FEV1.0 and vital capacity are decreased in both restrictive and obstructive diseases.
- The ratio of FEV1.0 to vital capacity is normal in restrictive disease but decreased in obstructive disease.

## 20.14. Pulmonary Function Testing

### 20.14.1. Pulmonary function testing, although rarely resulting in a diagnosis, is helpful in

1. Defining the type of process (obstruction and restriction) and the degree of functional impairment.
2. Following the course and treatment of disease.
3. Estimating the prognosis.
4. Preoperative evaluation.
5. Confirmation of functional impairment in patients having subjective complaints but a normal physical examination.

### 20.14.2. Spirometer and pulmonary function

- A spirometer is used to measure:
    - i. VC and its subdivisions
    - ii. Expiratory (or inspiratory) flow rates.

- Flow rates measured by spirometry usually include
    i.  FEV1
    ii.  Maximal midexpiratory flow rate.

### 20.14.3.  Restrictive diseases and pulmonary function

Restrictive diseases typically decrease
    i.  Total lung capacity (TLC)
    ii.  Vital capacity (VC).

### 20.14.4.  Obstructive diseases and pulmonary function

   i.  Increase residual volume and FRC.
  ii.  Peak expiratory flow is reduced in advanced obstructive disease.
 iii.  The forced expiratory volume in 1 sec (FEV1) correlates well with the severity of obstructive diseases.
  iv.  Maximal midexpiratory flow rate, the average flow during the middle 50% of the forced vital capacity (FVC), is a more reliable indicator of mild airway obstruction.
   v.  The flow rate at 25% VC (V25) is a useful index of small airway function.

### 20.15. The Most Common Causes of Epistaxis in Children

1.  Epistaxis digitorum  (nose picking).
2.  Trauma including child abuse.
3.  Foreign bodies.
4.  Medications (e.g. aspirin, anticoagulants, nonsteroidal anti-inflammatory drugs).
5.  Hypertension.
6.  Thrombocytopenia.

### 20.16. Condition that can Mimic the Common Cold

| Condition | Differentiating features |
|---|---|
| Allergic rhinitis | Prominent itching and sneezing |
|  | Nasal eosinophils |
| Foreign body | Unilateral, foul-smelling secretions |
|  | Bloody nasal secretions |
| Sinusitis | Presence of fever, headache or facial pain, or periorbital edema or persistence of rhinorrhea or cough for >14 days |

*Contd...*

*Contd...*

| Condition | Differentiating features |
|---|---|
| Streptococcosis | Mucopurulent nasal discharge that excoriates the nares |
| Pertussis | Onset of persistent or severe cough |
| Congenital syphilis | Persistent rhinorrhea with onset in the 1st 3 months of life |

## 20.17. Exercise-induced Bronchospasm

### 20.17.1. Sport activities that less likely than others to trigger exercise-induced bronchospasm

According to the American Academy of Allergy, Asthma and Immunology (AAAAI); Certain activities may be less likely than others to trigger exercise-induced bronchospasm:

- Swimming
- Walking
- Bike riding
- Hiking.

### 20.17.2. Symptoms of exercise-induced bronchospasm

- Shortness of breath or wheezing
- Decreased exercise endurance
- Chest pain or tightness with exercise
- Cough
- Upset stomach or stomachache
- Sore throat.

## 20.18. Lung Function Abnormalities in Asthma

Spirometry (in clinic):

    Airflow limitation:

        Low FEV1 (relative to percentage of predicted norms)

        FEV1/FVC ratio <0.80

    Bronchodilator response (to inhaled $\alpha$-agonist):

        Improvement in FEV1 $\geq$ 12% and $\geq$200 mL*

    Exercise challenge:

        Worsening in FEV1 $\geq$ 15%*

Daily peak flow or FEV1 monitoring: day to day and/or AM-to-PM variation $\geq$ 20%*

        *Main criteria consistent with asthma

    FEV1, forced expiratory volume in 1 sec; FVC and forced vital capacity

## 20.19. Lung Function Patterns (For Spirometry)

| Setting | Vital capacity | Peak flow | FEV1/ FVC | $MEF_{50}$ | $MIF_{50}$ |
|---|---|---|---|---|---|
| Poor effort/ weakness | Reduced | Reduced | Normal | Normal | Reduced |
| Mild asthma/cystic fibrosis | Normal | Normal | Normal | Reduced | Normal |
| Severe asthma/ cystic fibrosis | Reduced | Reduced | Reduced | Reduced | Normal |

## 20.20. Congenital Central Hypoventilation Syndrome (CCHS)

The clinical and physiological diagnosis of CCHS has been considered to require the following criteria

1.  Persistent evidence of hypoventilation during sleep

    [$PaCO_2 > 60$ mmHg (8 kPa)].

2.  Onset of symptoms usually in the first year after birth.

3.  Absence of primary pulmonary or neuromuscular disease.

4.  No evidence of primary heart disease.

## 20.21. Factors Suggesting Need for Hospitalization of Children with Pneumonia

1.  Age<6 months.

2.  Sickle cell anemia with acute chest syndrome.

3.  Multiple lobe involvement.

4.  Immunocompromised state.

5.  Toxic appearance.

6.  Moderate to severe respiratory distress.

7.  Requirement for supplemental oxygen.

8.  Dehydration.

9.  Vomiting or inability to tolerate oral fluids or medications.

10.  No response to appropriate oral antibiotic therapy   .

11.  Social factors (e.g. inability of caregivers to administer medications at home or follow up appropriately).

## 20.22. Differentiation of Pleural Fluid

|  | Transudate | Empyema |
|---|---|---|
| Appearance | Clear | Cloudy or purulent |
| Cell count (per mm$^3$) | <1000 | Often >50,000 (cell count has limited predictive value) |
| Cell type | Lymphocytes, monocytes | Polymorphonuclear leukocytes (neutrophils) |
| Lactate dehydrogenase | < 200 U/L | > 1000 U/L |
| Pleural fluid/serum LDH ratio | < 0.6 | > 0.6 |
| Protein >3 gm | Unusual | Common |
| Pleural fluid/serum protein ratio | < 0.5 | > 0.5 |
| Glucose | Normal | Low (< 40 mg/dL) |
| pH | Normal (7.40–7.60) | < 7.10 |
| Gram stain | Negative | Occasionally positive (less than one-third of cases) |

## 20.23. Low Glucose or pH in Pleural Fluid

Pleural fluid with low glucose or pH may be seen in:

- Malignant effusion
- Tuberculosis
- Esophageal rupture
- Pancreatitis (positive pleural amylase)
- Rheumatologic diseases (e.g. systemic lupus erythematosus).

## 20.24. Causes of Spontaneous Pneumothorax

### 20.24.1. Conditions associated with increased intrathoracic pressure

- Asthma
- Bronchiolitis
- Air-block syndrome in neonates
- Cystic fibrosis
- Airway foreign body.

### 20.24.2.  Congenital lung disease

- Congenital cystic adenomatoid malformation
- Bronchogenic cysts
- Pulmonary hypoplasia.

### 20.24.3.  Infection

- Pneumatocele
- Lung abscess
- Bronchopleural fistula.

### 20.24.4.  Diffuse lung disease

- Langerhans cell histiocytosis
- Tuberous sclerosis
- Marfan syndrome
- Ehlers-Danlos syndrome.

### 20.24.5.  Other conditions

- Primary idiopathic—Usually resulting from ruptured subpleural blebs
- Secondary blebs
- Metastatic neoplasm—Usually osteosarcoma (rare).

## 20.25. Cystic Fibrosis

### 20.25.1.  Respiratory symptoms may include the following

- Cough
- Recurrent wheezing
- Recurrent pneumonia
- Atypical asthma
- Dyspnea on exertion
- Chest pain.

### 20.25.2.  Gastrointestinal (GI) symptoms may include

- Meconium ileus
- Abdominal distension
- Intestinal obstruction
- Increased frequency of stools
- Failure to thrive (despite adequate appetite)
- Flatulence or foul-smelling flatus and steatorrhea
- Recurrent abdominal pain

- Jaundice
- GI bleeding.

### 20.25.3.  Genitourinary symptoms may include the following

- Undescended testicles or hydrocele
- Delayed secondary sexual development
- Amenorrhea.

### 20.25.4.  Pulmonary complications

- Bronchiectasis
- Atelectasis
- Pneumothorax
- Hemoptysis
- Hypertrophic pulmonary osteoarthropathy
- Allergic bronchopulmonary aspergillosis (ABPA)
- Pulmonary hypertension
- Cor pulmonale
- End-stage lung disease.

### 20.25.5.  Gastrointestinal complications

- Gastroesophageal reflux
- Meconium ileus
- Distal intestinal obstruction syndrome
- Rectal prolapse.

### 20.25.6.  Liver and pancreatic complications

- Fatty liver
- Focal biliary cirrhosis
- Portal hypertension
- Liver failure
- Cholecystitis and cholelithiasis
- Pancreatitis.

### 20.25.7.  Metabolic complications

- Vitamin deficiency (specially fat-soluble vitamins)
- Rickets
- Osteoporosis
- Cystic fibrosis-related diabetes mellitus.

### 20.25.8. Nasal complications

- Nasal polyps.
- Chronic and persistent sinusitis with complications such as mucopyocele formation.

## Bibliography


1. http://bentollenaar.com/_MM_Book/Ch.22.htm
2. http://emedicine.medscape.com/article/1001602-workup
3. http://emedicine.medscape.com/article/301914-overview
4. http://learnpediatrics.com/body-systems/respiratory-system/approach-to-pediatric-hemoptysis/
5. http://studynursing.blogspot.ae/2009/10/pulmonary-symptoms.html
6. http://www.clevelandclinicmeded.com/medicalpubs/diseasemanagement/pulmonary/pulmonary-function-testing/
7. http://www.webmd.com/lung/arthritis-sarcoidosis

# Rheumatology

## 21.1. Criteria for Diagnosis of Systemic Lupus Erythematosus (SLE)

**Note:** Must have at least 4 of 11.

1. Malar rash
2. Discoid rash
3. Photosensitivity
4. Oral ulcers
5. Arthritis
6. Serositis:
    i. Pleuritis
    ii. Pericarditis.
7. Renal disorder:
    i. Proteinuria
    ii. Cellular casts.
8. Neurologic disorder:
    i. Seizures
    ii. Psychosis.
9. Hematologic disorder:
    i. Hemolytic anemia
    ii. Leukopenia
    iii. Lymphopenia
    iv. Thrombocytopenia.
10. Immunologic disorder:
    i. Positive antiphospholipid ab
    ii. Anti-DNA ab
    iii. AntiSmith
    iv. False-positive syphilis test.
11. Antinuclear antibody.

## 21.2.  Common Presentation of Neonatal Lupus Erythematosus

- Rash
- Cytopenias
- Hepatitis
- Most importantly and congenital complete heart block.

## 21.3.  Diagnosis of Juvenile Dermatomyositis

- Presence of Heliotrope or Gottron Papules is required
- Plus at least 3 of the following 4 findings = Definite diagnosis
- Plus at least 2 of the following 4 findings = Probable diagnosis.

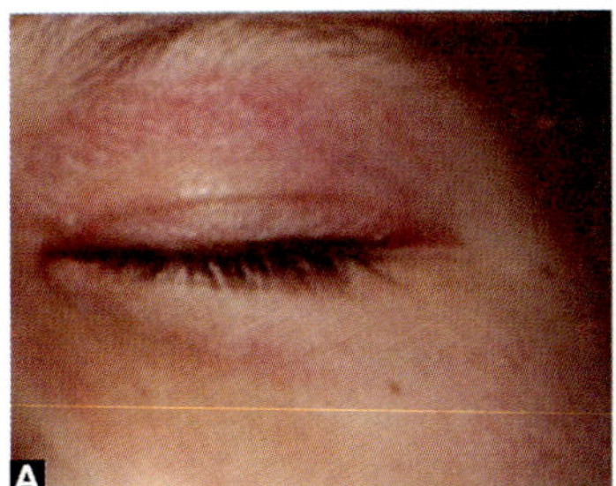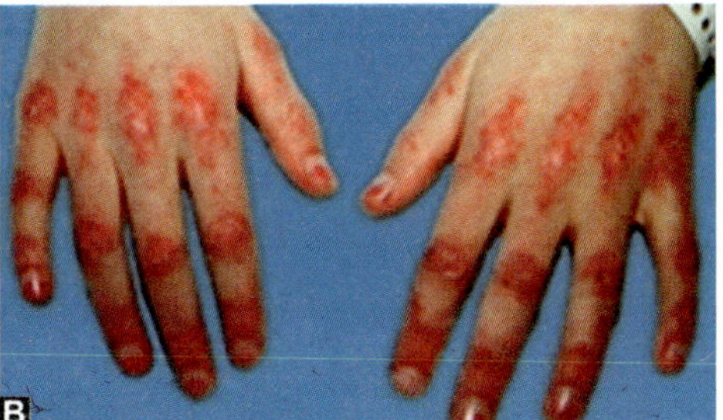

**Figs 21.1A and B**: Juvenile dermatomyositis

1. Symmetric proximal muscle
2. Elevated CPK, aldolase, LDH or transaminases
3. EMG abnormalities:
   a. Small amplitude, short duration and polyphasic motor-unit potentials.
   b. Fibrillations, positive sharp waves, increased insertional irritability.
   c. Spontaneous, bizarre high-frequency discharges.
4. Muscle biopsy abnormalities of:
   a. Degeneration
   b. Regeneration
   c. Necrosis
   d. Phagocytosis
   e. Interstitial mononuclear cell infiltrate.

## 21.4.  Kawasaki Disease

A clinical diagnosis requires fever for at least 5 days and a minimum of 4 of 5 findings:

1.  Bilateral conjunctivitis injection without exudates.
2.  Rash-usually macular, polymorphous with no vesicles, scaling or crusting in character on trunk and frequently more prominent in the perineal area later in the course, followed by desquamation of this area.
3.  Changes in lips and oral cavity—Red pharynx, dry fissured lips, or injected and strawberry tongue.
4.  Changes in the peripheral extremities—Edema  or redness of the hands/feet and later, desquamation of the fingers/toes.
5.  Cervical  lymphadenopathy—Usually  nonfluctuant  with  one  node required to be at least 1.5 cm in diameter.

## 21.5.  Systemic Juvenile Idiopathic Arthritis

### 21.5.1.  Poor prognostic indicators (3–6 months) of juvenile idiopathic arthritis

1.  Persistent fever
2.  Steroid dependency
3.  Thrombocytosis
4.  Polyarthritis
5.  Hip disease
6.  Early joint damage.

### 21.5.2.  High-spiking intermittent fever in systemic juvenile idiopathic arthritis

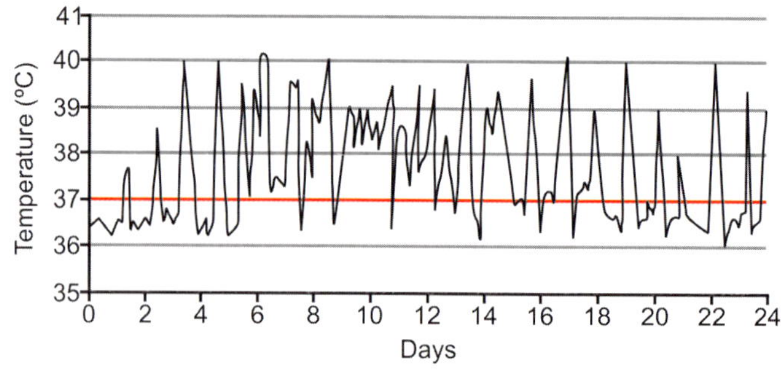


**Fig. 21.2**: Graph of fever in systemic juvenile idiopathic arthritis

## 21.6.  Characteristics Differentiation of the Spondyloarthritides

| Characteristic | Juvenile ankylosing spondylitis | Juvenile psoriatic arthritis | Inflammatory bowel disease | Reactive arthritis |
|---|---|---|---|---|
| Enthesitis | +++ | + | + | ++ |
| Axial arthritis | +++ | ++ | ++ | + |
| Peripheral arthritis | +++ | +++ | +++ | +++ |
| HLA-B27 positive | +++ | + | +++ | +++ |
| Antinuclear antibody positive | – | ++ | – | – |
| Rheumatoid factor positive | – | – | – | – |
| Systemic disease: | | | | |
|   Eyes | + | + | + | + |
|   Skin | – | – | + | + |
|   Mucous membranes | – | – | + | + |
|   Gastrointestinal tract | – | – | ++++ | ++++ |

*Frequency of characteristics*:
   –: absent; + :<25%; ++: 25–50%; +++: 50–75%, ++++: 75% or more

## 21.7.  Viruses Associated with Arthritis

### 21.7.1.  Herpesviruses

1.  Epstein-Barr
2.  Cytomegalovirus
3.  Varicella zoster
4.  Herpes simplex.

### 21.7.2.  Enteroviruses

1.  Echovirus
2.  Coxsackievirus B.

### 21.7.3.  Hepadnavirus

Hepatitis B.

### 21.7.4. Paramyxoviruses

Mumps.

### 21.7.5. Adenoviruses

Adenovirus 7.

### 21.7.6. Orthopoxviruses

1. Variola virus (smallpox)
2. Vaccinia virus.

### 21.7.7. Togaviruses

#### *21.7.7.1. Rubivirus*

Rubella.

#### *21.7.7.2. α-viruses*

1. Ross river
2. Chikungunya
3. O'nyong-nyong
4. Mayaro
5. Sindbis
6. Ockelbo
7. Pogosta.

### 21.7.8. Parvoviruses

## 21.8. Morbidity in Childhood Lupus

| System | Morbidity |
| --- | --- |
| Renal | Hypertension, dialysis and transplantation |
| Central nervous system | Organic brain syndrome, seizures, psychosis and neurocognitive dysfunction |
| Cardiovascular | Atherosclerosis, myocardial infarction, cardiomyopathy and valvular disease |
| Immune | Recurrent infection, functional asplenia and malignancy |
| Musculoskeletal | Osteopenia, compression fractures and osteonecrosis |
| Ocular | Cataracts and glaucoma |
| Endocrine | Diabetes, obesity, growth failure, infertility and fetal wastage |

## 21.9.  Definition of Arthritis

Arthritis is defined by intra-articular swelling or the presence of 2 or more of the following signs:
1.  Limitation in range of motion
2.  Tenderness or pain on motion
3.  Increased heat or erythema.

## 21.10. Arthralgias without Physical Findings for Arthritis

Arthralgias without physical findings for arthritis suggest:
1.  Infection
2.  Malignancy
3.  Orthopedic conditions
4.  Benign syndromes, or pain syndromes such as fibromyalgia.

## 21.11. Arthritis as a Presenting Manifestation of Multisystem Rheumatic  Diseases of Childhood

1.  Systemic lupus erythematosus
2.  Juvenile dermatomyositis
3.  Sarcoidosis
4.  Vasculitic syndromes.

## 21.12. Symptoms Characteristic of Inflammatory Back Pain

1.  Pain at night with morning stiffness
2.  No improvement with rest
3.  Improvement with exercise
4.  Insidious onset.

## 21.13. Reactive Arthritis

Reactive arthritis typically follows:
  i.  Enteric infection with:
1.  *Salmonella*
2.  *Shigella*
3.  *Yersinia enterocolitica*
4.  *Campylobacter jejuni*
5.  *Cryptosporidium parvum*
6.  *Giardia intestinalis.*
  ii.  Genitourinary tract infection with:
1.  *Chlamydia trachomatis*
2.  *Ureaplasma.*

## 21.14. Drug-induced Lupus

### 21.14.1. Definit association

1. Adalimumab
2. Chlorpromazine
3. Etanercept
4. Diltiazem
5. Hydralazine
6. Infliximab, interferon and isoniazid
7. Methyldopa and minocycline
8. Penicillamine and procainamide.

### 21.14.2. Probable association

1. Amiodarone
2. β-blockers
3. Captopril and carbamazepine
4. Docetaxel
5. Ethosuximide
6. Gemfibrozil, glyburide, gold and griseofulvin
7. Hydrochlorothiazide
8. Interferon-γ
9. Lithium
10. Nitrofurantoin
11. Penicillin, phenytoin and propylthiouracil
12. Quinidine
13. Rifampin
14. Statins and sulfasalazine
15. Tetracycline
16. Valproate.

### 21.14.3. Facts about drug-induced lupus

1. These agents may act as a trigger for true SLE.
2. These agents provoke a reversible lupus-like syndrome.
3. Drug-induced lupus affects males and females equally.
4. An inherited predisposition toward slow acetylation may increase the risk of drug-induced lupus.

5. Circulating antihistone antibodies are often present in drug-induced SLE, and these antibodies are detected in upto 20% of individuals with SLE.
6. Hepatitis, which is rare in SLE, is more common in drug-induced lupus.
7. Individuals with drug-induced lupus are less likely to demonstrate:
    i. Antibodies to double-stranded DNA
    ii. Hypocomplementemia
    iii. Significant renal or neurologic disease.
8. Manifestations of drug-induced lupus resolve after withdrawal of the offending medication.
9. Complete recovery may take several months to years.

## 21.15. The Screening Musculoskeletal Examination in a Child

1. Extend the arms straight out in front then make a fist.
2. Place palms and fingers together with wrists extended to 90°: 'Prayer position'.
3. Raise arms straight above the head.
4. Turn neck to look over each shoulder.
5. Walk normally, on tip-toe and on the heels.
6. Sit cross-legged on the floor then jump up.

*A child who can perform all these actions without difficulty is unlikely to have a significant musculoskeletal problem.*

## 21.16. Causes of Migratory Arthritis

1. Gonococcal arthritis
2. Rheumatic fever
3. Sarcoidosis
4. Systemic lupus erythematosus
5. Lyme disease
6. Bacterial endocarditis
7. Whipple's disease.

## 21.17. Causes of Polyarthritis

### 21.17.1. Causes of symmetric polyarthritis

1. Rheumatoid arthritis
2. Systemic lupus erythematosus
3. Psoriatic arthritis
4. Osteoarthritis
5. Scleroderma

6. Lyme disease
7. Rheumatic fever
8. Gouty arthritis
9. Pseudogout
10. Liver disease.

## 21.17.2. Causes of asymmetric polyarthritis

1. Spondyloarthropathy (HLA-B27 disease)
    i. Psoriatic arthritis
    ii. Ankylosing spondylitis
    iii. Reactive arthritis
    iv. Inflammatory bowel disease.
2. Gouty arthritis
3. Pseudogout
4. Lyme disease
5. Viral arthritis.

## 21.18. Henoch-Schönlein Purpura (HSP)

### 21.18.1. HSP symptoms

Symptoms: Classic triad (beyond rash, triad is not uniformly present)
1. Palpable purpuric rash on lower extremities
2. Abdominal pain or renal involvement (nephritis)
3. Arthritis.

### 21.18.2. HSP signs

1. Rash (100% of cases)
2. Abdominal pain (60–80% of cases)
3. Joint involvement (70% of cases)
4. Renal disease (25–50% of cases).

### 21.18.3. HSP complications (more common in adults)

#### 21.18.3.1. Cardiopulmonary conditions

1. Myocardial infarction
2. Pulmonary hemorrhage
3. Pleural effusion.

### *21.18.3.2. Gastrointestinal conditions*

1. Intussusception (mural hematoma is lead point) in 5% of cases
2. Gastrointestinal bleeding
3. Bowel infarction.

### *21.18.3.3. Neurologic conditions*

1. Seizures
2. Mononeuropathies.

### *21.18.3.4. Renal disorders*

1. Crescentic glomerulonephritis
2. Renal failure
3. Hematuria
4. Proteinuria.

### *21.18.3.5. Male genitourinary conditions*

1. Orchitis
2. Testicular torsion.

## Bibliography


1. http://emedicine.medscape.com/article/1006582-medication
2. http://www.fpnotebook.com/HemeOnc/Derm/HnchSchnlnPrpr.htm
3. http://www.fpnotebook.com/Rheum/joint/PlyrtclrArthrts.htm
4. http://www.medicinenet.com/kawasaki_disease/article.htm
5. http://www.rheumatology.org/Practice/Clinical/Patients/Diseases_And_ Conditions/Dermatomyositis_%28Juvenile%29/
6. http://www.the-rheumatologist.org/details/article/2041587/Systemic_ Juvenile_Idiopathic_Arthritis.html

# Pediatric Mnemonics

## 22.1.  APGAR Score Components

**APGAR:**

Appearance: Cyanosis—Peripheral, central and none
Pulse: Pulse rate
Grimace: Response to stimulation
Activity: Movement of the baby (muscle tone)
Respiration: Respiratory rate.

## 22.2.  Autistic Disorder: Features

**AUTISTICS:**

**A**gain and again (repetitive behavior)
**U**nusual abilities
**T**alking (language) delay
**I**Q subnormal
**S**ocial development poor
**T**hree years onset
**I**nherited component [35% concordance]
**C**ognitive impairment
**S**elf-injury.

## 22.3.  Breastfeeding: Contraindicated Drugs

**BREAST:**

**B**romocriptine/**B**enzodiazepines
**R**adioactive isotopes/**R**izatriptan
**E**rgotamine/**E**thosuximide
**A**miodarone/**A**mphetamines
**S**timulant laxatives/**S**ex hormones
**T**etracycline/**T**retinoin.

## 22.4. Branches of Facial Nerve

Ten Zebras Beat My Cock
Temporal, Zygomatic, Buccal, Mandibular and Cervical.

## 22.5. Cyanotic Congenital Heart Diseases

**5 T's:**
Truncus arteriosus
Transposition of the great arteries
Tricuspid atresia
Tetralogy of Fallot
Total anomalous pulmonary venous return.

## 22.6. ECG: T Wave Inversion Causes

**INVERT:**
Ischemia
Normality [specially young and black]
Ventricular hypertrophy
Ectopic foci [e.g. calcified plaques]
RBBB and LBBB
Treatments [digoxin].

## 22.7. Innocent Murmurs

**S$_3$LAC:**
Soft
Systolic
Short
Left sternal age
Asymptomatic
Change with posture.

## 22.8. Meckel's Diverticulum-Rule of 2's

**2** inches long
**2** feet from the ileocecal valve
**2**% of the population
Commonly presents in the first 2 years of life may contain **2** types of epithelial tissue.

## 22.9.    Murmurs: Questions to Ask

**SCRIPT**:
Site
Character (e.g. harsh, soft, blowing)
Radiation
Intensity
Pitch
Timing.

## 22.10. Murmurs: Innocent Murmur Features.8 S's

Soft
Systolic
Short
Sounds (S1 and S2) normal
Symptomless
Special tests normal (X-ray and EKG)
Standing/Sitting (vary with position)
Sternal depression.

## 22.11. Paramyxoviruses Family

$PRM_3$
Parainfluenza
Respiratory syncytial virus
Mumps
Measles
Metapneumovirus.

## 22.12. Pheochromocytoma-rule of 10%s

**10%** malignant
**10%** bilateral
**10%** extra-adrenal
**10%** calcified
**10%** children
**10%** familial.

## 22.13. Potter Syndrome

**POTTER**:
**P**ulmonary hypoplasia
**O**ligohydramnios
**T**wisted skin (wrinkly skin)
**T**wisted face (Potter facies)
**E**xtremities defects
**R**enal agenesis (bilateral).

## 22.14. Protein Content of Milk

Human: 1.1
Cow: 2.2
Buffalo: 3.3
Goat :4.4.

## 22.15. Psoriasis: Pathophysiology

**PSORIASIS**:
**P**ink **P**apules/**P**laques/**P**inpoint bleeding (Auspitz sign)/**P**hysical injury (Koebner phenomenon)/**P**ain.
**S**ilver scale/**S**harp margins.
**O**nycholysis/**O**il spots.
**R**ete Ridges with **R**egular elongation.
**I**tching.
**A**rthritis/**A**bscess (Munro).
**S**tratum corneum with nuclei and neutrophils.
**I**mmunologic.
**S**tratum granulosum absent/**S**tratum spinosum thickening.

## 22.16. Radial Nerve Innervates the BEST!!!!

**B**rachioradialis
**E**xtensors
**S**upinator
**T**riceps.

## 22.17. Rash Appearance in a Febrile Patient

"Really Sick Children Must Try Duck Eggs"
1st day: **R**ubella
2nd day: **S**carlet fever/**S**mallpox
3rd day: **C**hickenpox (1–5 days)
4th day: **M**easles (Koplik spots seen a day prior to the rash)
5th day: **T**yphus and **R**ickettsia (this is variable)
6th day: **D**engue (**M**orbilliform, over dorsum of hands and feet; trunk)
7th day: **E**nteric fever (**R**ose spots over abdomen, flanks and back).

## 22.18. Risk Factor for Neonatal Jaundice

**JAUNDICE:**
**J**aundice within 24 hours
**A** sibling with jaundice
**U**nrecognized hemolysis
**N**onoptimal sucking
**D**eficiency of G6PD
**I**nfection
**C**ephalhematoma
**E**ast Asia.

## 22.19. Raynaud's Phenomenon: Causes

**COLD HAND:**
**C**ryoglobulins/**C**ryofibrinogens
**O**bstruction/**O**ccupational
**L**upus erythematosus, other connective tissue disease
**D**iabetes mellitus/**D**rugs
**H**ematologic problems (polycythemia, leukemia, etc.)
**A**rterial problems (atherosclerosis)
**N**eurologic problems (vascular tone)
**D**isease of unknown origin (idiopathic).

## 22.20. STURGE Weber

**STURGE**
**S**eizures
**T**rigeminal port-wine stain

Unilateral weakness (often opposite side to stain)
Retardation (mental) in some patients
Glaucoma
Eye problems, e.g. buphthalmos.

## 22.21. White Patch of Skin: Differential

"Vitiligo **PATCH**":
**V**itiligo
**P**ityriasis alba/**P**ostinflammatory hypopigmentation
**A**ge-related hypopigmentation
**T**inea versicolor/**T**uberous sclerosis (ash leaf macule)
**C**ongenital birthmark
**H**ansen's (leprosy).

## 22.22. Williams Syndrome

**WILLIAMS**
**W**eight (low at birth and slow to gain)
**I**ris (stellate iris)
**L**ong philtrum
**L**arge mouth
**I**ncreased $Ca^{++}$
**A**ortic stenosis (and other stenosis)
**M**ental retardation
**S**welling around eyes (periorbital puffiness).

## 22.23. DiGeorge Syndrome

**CATCH-22**:
**C**ongenital heart disease
**A**bnormal facies
**T**hymic aplasia
**C**left palate
**H**ypocalcemia
**22**q deletion

## 22.24. Short Stature

Short stature: differential **ABCDEFG**:
**A**lone (neglected infant)

Bone dysplasias (rickets, scoliosis and mucopolysaccharidoses)
Chromosomal (Turner's and Down's)
Delayed growth
Endocrine (low growth hormone, Cushing's and hypothyroid)
Familial
GI malabsorption (celiac and Crohn's).

## 22.25. Breastfeeding: Contraindicated Drugs BREAST

Bromocriptine/Benzodiazepines
Radioactive isotopes/Rizatriptan
Ergotamine/Ethosuximide
Amiodarone/Amphetamines
Stimulant laxatives/Sex hormones
Tetracycline/Tretinoin.

## 22.26. Congenital Adrenal Hyperplasia (CAH)

**Congenital Adrenal Hyperplasia (CAH)**: Endocrine, congenital, most common. Mnemonic: One up! first number refers to aldosterone, second number to Testosterone. If that number is one then that hormone is elevated. 21-Hydroxylase (most common!), 17-Hydroxylase, 11-Hydroxylase, 3-Hydroxylase

| A–T | Aldosterone | Cortisol | Testosterone |
|-----|-------------|----------|--------------|
| 2–1 | Low | Low | Elevated |
| 1–7 | Elevated | Low | Low |
| 1–1 | Elevated | Low | Elevated |
| 0–3 | Low | Low | Low |

And remember this tells you the symptoms too. ↑Aldosterone if elevated leads to hypertension, hypokalemia. ↑Testosterone if elevated in females leads to virilizing often at birth. Shows up later in males.

## 22.27. Causes of Elevated Anion Gap Metabolic Acidosis

**MUDPILES**
Methanol
Uremia (renal failure)
Diabetic, alcoholic or starvation ketoacidosis
Paracetamol, propylene glycol, paregoric

Inborn errors of metabolism, iron, ibuprofen and isoniazid

Lactic acid

Ethylene glycol

Salicylates (aspirin)s.

## 22.28. Causes of Normal Anion Gap Metabolic Acidosis

**DR. C**

Diarrhea.

Renal tubular acidosis type I, II, IV (hypoaldosteronism) or medication induced.

Chloride excess (from saline fluid resuscitation, hyperalimentation, or increased gastrointestinal $Cl^-$ reabsorption from fistulae or ureteral diversion).

## 22.29. Causes of Respiratory Alkalosis

**AMISH**

Ammonia (urea cycle defect and hepatic encephalopathy), anxiety

Medications (progesterone and salicylates)

Increased intracranial pressure

Sepsis

Hypoxemia and hyperthermia.

## 22.30. Measles: Complications "MEASLES COMP" (Complications)

Myocarditis

Encephalitis

Appendicitis

Subacute sclerosing panencephalitis

Laryngitis

Early death

Shits (diarrhea)

Corneal ulcer

Otitis media

Mesenteric lymphadenitis

Pneumonia and related (bronchiolitis-bronchitis-croup).

## Bibliography


1. http://medmnemonics.wordpress.com/category/paediatrics/
2. http://theweeklymnemonic.wordpress.com/category/surgery/pediatric/
3. http://worldofmedicalmnemonics.blogspot.ae/2008/08/pediatric-mnemonics.html
4. http://www.lifehugger.com/pediatrics?page=7
5. http://www.medicalmnemonics.com/cgi-bin/return_browse.cfm?discipline=Pediatrics&browse=1
6. http://www.rxpgonline.com/modules.php?name=Mnemonics&func=CatView&cat=5
7. http://www.valuemd.com/pediatrics_mnemonics.php

# Suggested Reading


1. Kliegman Robert M, Behrman Richard E. Nelson Textbook of Pediatrics. 19th ed.(revision).
2. Megan M. Tschudy, Kristin M. Arcara. The Harriet Lane handbook . 19th ed. Johns Hopkins Hospital.Children's Medical and Surgical Center. (revision).
3. Neil Mclntosh, Peter Helms. Forfar and Arneil's Textbook of Pediatrics.7th ed (revision).
4. Thomas CJ, Robert AH. Common Pediatric Problems; Pediatric Board Review Core Curriculum. 4th ed. Medstay 2010-2011. Colorado

# Index